The
WEIGHT LOSS CHALLENGE

Brenda Boddy

To my wonderful Husband.
Thank you for believing in me, for being supportive, and for accepting me for who I am. Your continual love pulls me through any self doubt and gives me the strength to reach for the stars. I am blessed to spend my life with a man, who I not only love, but respect.

To my Children.
You have all grown into so much more than offspring…you are also my best friends. Because of you I kept trying to get my fitness right, struggling back on track, when I really wanted to just bag it. I so much wanted to be a good example to you. You have all put up with years of my pushing to exercise, tasted my crazy recipes as I looked for healthy substitutions to basic meals, and listened to my (dare I admit?) nagging to buy whole foods instead of processed. At every turn in my life you have been there, supporting me with your love and I will never be able to express adequately how much each one of you mean to me and how proud I am of the young adults you have become.

To my Parents.
It was because of you I have so many of my values. You have taught me the importance of good work ethics, instilled in me the belief that I can do anything, and shared, through example, how love for one another can take you through any obstacles life throws at you. I will always love you.

INTRODUCTION

I have always struggled with my weight. One of my best friends in high school was a very slender Vietnamese/American girl, and I can remember early on trying to diet my curvy American body down to be as small as she was, not taking into account different ethnic looks and body styles. I soon worked myself into eating disorders, diet mentality (If I break the diet today, I will eat everything I can because I'll be depriving myself tomorrow.), and bouts of depression and hopelessness that follows with weight gain and low self-esteem.

I spent a decade weeping and despairing over my weight as I tried every diet and pill. It was a long journey to realize that it was not about spending money on the next magic gimmick, but doing the work.

I became a fitness trainer, thinking that if I immersed myself in the lifestyle, I would become lean. I learned to love exercise and creating programs to help others get fit. I felt blessed to be able to help those who were dealing with injuries and muscle imbalances become strong and fit.

Still, I continued to have nutrition issues for myself. I felt like a failure. My own weight would yo yo up and down. My self confidence was at the bottom.

In June 2013, we started a weight loss challenge in our gym. As an employee I was not eligible to do the challenge, but I began a blog to help others work through their weight loss journey.

My thought behind starting the blog was, "I have years of nutrition and exercise education that I have rambling around in my head, but I have never put it together in a way that helps me when I am feeling weak." So every day I tried to take an area of fitness to blog about in a way that might help others who were struggling. Often this was the very area I was struggling with or needed reminding myself about. The hour or so it took me to put my thoughts down, reinforced my own forward momentum and helped me think about my choices for the day. Little by little I start to evolve myself. I began changing from the outside in, about how I viewed myself.

I now accept that I am not perfect. I recognize that I am a child of the creator and am blessed. I know that I am walking my own journey and will arrive at my destination at the time that is right for me. The reality was that I set out to help others and ended up helping myself.

The Weight Loss Challenge Book is a tool to help you reach your own goals. Read the daily blog no matter how well or bad you do each day. Then journal your own thoughts and progress notes about your day. Use whatever nutrition and exercise program best suits you.

When you finish the 8 weeks, restart the program. Good attitudes and progress comes with repeated exposure and practice. For most of us the journey is not always easy. I've found it is worth it.

BEFORE YOU BEGIN

I'm not here to tell you which diet to use or how to exercise. This is your challenge.

Have you ever had a friend tell you about a great diet that they found and lost mega weight on? Then when you tried the diet, you felt like a failure? That's because we are all unique and walk a different path. We all have a different lifestyle and so different diets work for different people depending on habits concerning when they eat and types of food that they like, along with what their individual triggers are.

You aren't a failure. You are different than anyone else, so it is important for you to choose a LIFESTYLE of eating that merges with your own style. Weight loss is about calories in/calories out. But how, when, and where you consume those calories will determine your success. Choose your plan wisely so that it is a way of life that can be sustained, and not a diet that you will ultimately fall off.

Create a vision board to make your goals real in your head. When you can 'SEE' where you are going, you know where you are going.

Plan when you are going to eat, where you are going to eat, how often you are going to eat, and what you are going to eat.

Plan when, where, how, and how often you are going to exercise.

Commit yourself to jump back in the game, whether you run your race perfectly or stumble occasionally. Successful people just dust themselves off and get back on board.

Try to take multiple numbers and measurements of where you are when you start. This would be things like physical measurements of basic body parts (chest, waist, etc.), fat percentage, muscle percentage, and weight. A before picture is also a great tool.

This way you know where you are coming from. If you have a week when you seem to plateau, you can see that maybe your muscle percentage went up or your inches went down.

Believe in yourself.

DAY 1

Good Morning!
Working on that challenge today? So let's get real. Do you have a plan? Because if you are drifting along hoping this is enough motivation to get that weight off and you have not come up with a better way of living, you are going to end up with the same old results.

Visualize where you are going. Make sure you have a nutrition plan set out. PACK those meals and snacks that you plan to eat, and the times you will eat them, so that you aren't tempted to reach for something that's not nutritious. Plan when you will exercise and what you will do. Then take action. Remember how lousy you have felt while heavy, how embarrassed, how awkward and unable to follow your dreams. This is your chance. Put your vision in front of you and go for it!

DAY 2

Good morning.

So did you follow your plan yesterday? Because a dream is only a dream, unless you take action. Did you have trouble packing your nutrition in the morning? Then try packing it the night before. Or cook on the weekend. Which brings us today's point. FAIL FAST. If what you are doing isn't working then change your plan of action immediately and find something that does. We wouldn't start a journey across country without a roadmap, but we'll meander along on our fitness path hoping to get to our destination.

And quit making excuses. You say you didn't have time to pack your nutrition, but you had time to grab that donut. You had time to sit on the couch and eat a half bag of chips while watching TV. Nobody held a gun to your head and made you eat a second or third helping instead of going for a walk. When you take responsibility for where you are and the choices you make, then you can make choices to transform yourself.

You were created with unlimited potential. Somewhere along the way you've quit believing in yourself. You have to live in your body and with yourself the rest of your life. Stop allowing circumstances, others, and lack of commitment to steal your power. When you take responsibility for the choices you make, you take back your power, remove those mountains from in front of you, and begin your transformation back to health.

DAY 3

Good morning.
It's going to be a great day! What's that you say? "I have a bummer schedule at work today. I'm out of energy today. I'm dreading my chore list today. I look terrible in this outfit...I can't stay on a diet...Look how fat my arms are....I'll never look as good as that coworker looks..." Have you been listening to yourself lately? Our destiny is coming out of our own minds. We will say ugly, nasty things to ourselves that we would never say to anyone else. And your mind believes it. If you are saying you can never lose weight, you are locking yourself into an overweight, unhealthy, and hopeless feeling that is a result of what you believe. Your body is just doing what you are telling it. For many of us, that towering mountain that has been in our way is the one we put there ourselves, when we quit believing in what we are capable us.

We need to start speaking out loud our path of transformation. "I CAN EAT HEALTHY AND EXERCISE EVERY DAY...I have the ability to transform myself....My body feels energized when I put nutritious food in it...I am getting fitter and stronger daily...I have the best attitude at work...I am able to manage my budget...I am a good spouse (helpful coworker, great dad, etc.). Every time you speak a negative thought into your life, you are adding another log of burden that weighs you down. But when you speak blessing in your life, your mind believes that also. Your self-esteem comes up. You begin to believe in your own worth and ability to change. And guess what? Your body and lifestyle begins to change to match what you believe.

Pay attention to your inner dialogue and counter it with affirmative thoughts spoken out loud. You DO have the ability to lose weight and get fit. You have the power and control to change. It's up to you.

DAY 4

Good morning.
Still have your eyes set on that transformation you are achieving? Beyond having a plan of action, you need to be able to see the end result. One person told me they were already planning the dress they will wear on vacation when they are at their weight goal. That's a part of visualizing the final result.

How many of us have lost weight and then gained it (or more) back? I would encourage everyone to take a picture of your self to compare to your end results. I know ...I know...most of us avoid mirrors like they were the enemy. Or when we stand in the mirror, we hold our belly in and admire ourselves from our best angle. Unfortunately that is not always the picture others see. When we take a photo (front, back, and sides) it is a realistic blueprint of what we need to build on; Are your shoulders rounded over? You need to strengthen your upper back (rhomboids) and stretch your chest area to allow your posture to return to normal. Feet turn out? Your inner thighs need strengthening to pull your feet back into alignment, and your outer legs need stretched to quit pulling outward so strongly. And I can't emphasize enough that if you are having shoulder, knee or back pain that you need to be in a corrective exercise program.

You work a fixed amount of your life. But you live in your body 24 hours a day, every day, for as long as you live. This challenge is not only about losing weight, but bringing your temple, your body, back into alignment with what it was meant to be. You are awesomely created and your body is meant to be an active asset to live your life at your highest potential. You don't want to throw that gift away.

After you have taken your picture, find a picture of what you want your end result to look like. (You can even go so far as to paste your head on the body of who you want to look like). So many of us have been heavy and out of shape so long that we have trouble envisioning what we could be. Make sure the picture you choose is realistic. (The picture you choose should have the same body height and structure. If you are 4 foot, your head should not be pasted on top of a 6 foot model).

After the first shock of looking at your new after picture, your mind will start to adjust to that new look. You now have something to envision when you are pushing yourself to do that extra half mile, or stay up another 15 minutes to pack your lunch.

Everyday can be the best day of your life. Choose to live it with passion. Put a smile on your face and tell yourself how much you love life and your journey.

DAY 5

Good morning.

Do you pick up an article about weight loss or health and read the same old information...blah, blah, set goals, blah, blah, make a vision board, blah...and quit reading? Most people know they should follow through and do this, but never take the time to actually do it. We really are looking for the article that tells us about the next great break through; preferably a pill that will make us skinny, pack on muscle, bring prosperity, and success.

The reason we set goals and make a vision board is to take us to the most important step in transforming ourselves. We bring our vision to life by the words we speak out loud where our ears can hear. When you wake up, your vision board uses your sense of sight to imagine your goals, but your voice activates those dreams. When you speak blessings and favor into your life, you direct your destiny.

A person who starts their day by saying, "I am powerful. I am prosperous. Money comes to me easily. I am successful. I can run my own business. People like me. I have great work ethics. I love my job and rise to the top", will find their careers moving forward through their faith.

The person who says, "I am free from my addictions. I have the power to make good nutritional choices. Food that is processed and full of sugar and unhealthy fat is repulsive to me and I only crave healthy, wholesome choices of lean meat, fruit, vegetables, and dairy," will eventually see a transforming inside themselves toward their goals as their mind recreates who they believe they are. Even when you are picking up that doughnut, you need to speak, out loud, your disgust for what sugar does to your body and energy. One day you will reach past the doughnut and grab the apple

The person who says, " I love to exercise. I find an opportunity to exercise everyday. I make appointments with myself to exercise. I find new ways to exercise to make it fun. My body is getting leaner and stronger every day. I never allow myself to make excuses to skip my exercise. I am powerful and strong and sexy and getting younger every day.", will realize that at some point they have become what they are saying every day.

This works in the opposite way. When someone asks you how you are, do you bring out your list of ailments? "I'm fine, but I just hate my job. I can't seem to shake my cold. I catch everything that comes along. I always seem to be tired and out of energy" Listen to what you are saying because this is what you will be even more of in five years.

Do you call four friends and tell them how frustrated you are at your spouse, how depressed you are at being in debt, how fat and dejected you are, how badly your kids misbehave? Take a look at what you are talking about, because you are pulling even more of that into your life. Your ears are listening to you being depressed, whiny, and feeling like a loser. If you feel bad now, you are going to feel even worse in a few years when your marriage is worse, you are heavier and more depressed, you have a bad relationship with your kids, and you are at the bottom of your boss's favor list.

Love your self and appreciate the blessing of being alive. You have value and a unique combination of talents that nobody else has. Take the time to set your goals and create your vision board to remind yourself to speak those things into your life daily. When you believe something to be good and true about yourself, your body and environment will change to be in alignment with your belief.

Day 6

Good morning.
You are at the end of your first week now. KEEP GOING.
Humans make mistakes, underestimate, overestimate,
and fall short. We also reach peaks of performance that
no other life form on earth has the capability to reach.
Learn from your journey and tweak your plan, but never
give up. You didn't like where you were at the beginning
of the week, and you will like it even less if you stop
trying.

In America we eat for many reasons, most of them
having little to do with genuine hunger or nourishment
for our bodies. Our emotions are often our driving force
behind what we choose, and when we choose to eat. Pay
attention to why you want to eat, and then look at your
body language when you feel that way.

Example: Someone says something and it makes you
feel bad. You don't want to be ugly back so you stuff
down your anger and immediately feel like eating
something unhealthy. Eating satisfies a need in you.
When you zone out and eat something sweet and/or
fatty, that wonderful first few bites gives you a surge of
pleasure. And you are in control of what you grab.
Others can make you angry, but they can't stop you
from eating something that feels good.

Example: you are working on your fitness and you see some really cute, trim person. Your inner dialogue immediately says, "I will never look like that". So you are depressed. When you are feeling down and out, that yummy first few bites of something full of sugar and fat not only gives you a great taste sensation, but the fast entry of sugar into your system raises your blood sugar and gives you (temporarily) more energy. Of course, you crash fairly fast and now your body is on a yo-yo to keep eating in order to recapture that energy burst. You are chasing the sugar drug. Think about it. Cocaine is a plant that is processed into a fine white addictive powder. Sugar is a plant that is processed into a fine white addictive powder. See the connection?

The thing to focus on is that emotions are often fairly fleeting. When you are depressed you think similar thoughts (I am ugly, I feel useless and out of energy, I always fail when I diet). You put your body into a familiar stance (your shoulders slump, your actions slow, your mouth turns down, you dwell on your unhappy thoughts) Your body and emotions mimics your thought pattern and you finish by going to your food drug of choice to numb yourself and get through your depressive attitude. Although you feel better immediately when you eat sugary/fat food, you will later begin to chastise yourself for your lack of control and willpower. Your negative self-dialogue throws you back into anger and depression and the cycle of reaching for the sugar drug begins again.

We have choices! When you find your emotions going negative through something or someone who affects us, we can immediately use our emotions on the opposite side of the scale. Straighten your shoulders, put your head back, and smile. Think of a time or instance that made you feel super excited and happy, (birth of a child, intimate moment, wedding, graduation, etc.) Begin speaking out positive affirmations to yourself (I am strong, I have choices, I am getting fitter every moment, my body is unique and changing to meet the new me, I don't have to compete with anyone else, I have the power to make healthy choices and others cannot force me to be unhealthy). Follow your action plan with something small and nourishing and follow through with lots of water. Find something interesting to do.

I cannot emphasize enough that you are in a transformation. As soon as your mind makes the choice to change, you are a new person, not subject to your old addictions and habits. It just takes a while for your body to catch up to the new you. Like the sluggish caterpillar that is in the cocoon, you are moving toward a fabulous finish. Every time you eat something healthy, pack a meal ahead of schedule, or exercise intensely, you are putting the sluggish caterpillar further in your past, and stretching your wing to break out into a new you. Enjoy the journey and the new lessons you are teaching yourself. No one in the world, of billions of people, is as unique or wonderful as you. You are fearfully and wonderfully created, and your creator NEVER creates garbage! Your eyes are opening to the many great adventures you are going to have in a fit body with unlimited potential.

DAY 7

Good morning.

Remember that our routines change on the weekend. Now is an important time to really plan those meals around your events so that you stay on track. An entire week of hard effort can be derailed with lack of preparation. And you did not like how you felt before you started this fitness journey, so don't allow yourself to go there again.

Some people allow themselves a cheat meal or cheat day. But be real...you know yourself. If you haven't got a plan of action for those times when you are not in a structured setting (birthday parties, family gatherings, working in the yard and eating on the run, etc.), then your plan is to fail. You will do what you've always done. How successful was your fitness with that routine? And if a cheat meal is going to lead to a cheat day which is going to lead to a cheat week, then you will be better off staying on track until you have firmly established a lifestyle of reaching for nutritious choices in the right amount for your body's needs.

DAY 8

Good morning.

Kudos to those who did well on their nutrition this week. If you didn't, NOW is the time to get back into gear. You liked how your felt when you started this challenge...hopeful, excited, moving forward. You hated how you felt before you started this challenge...disgusted, embarrassed, depressed, out of energy. Use that painful emotion, you felt, to figure out how to fix your plan and move onward.

When you started your journey, we talked about matching your nutrition plan to your lifestyle. Let's look at this closer.

For example: You habitually eat munchies when you work on the computer. A diet that asks you to eat three meals a day at the table, with no snacks, will be difficult for you. Instead, substitute in foods that are healthier at the computer (veggies, unbuttered popcorn, etc.)

Diets also specify foods that may not be favorites of everyone. Look at your chosen nutrition plan ahead of time and substitute in foods that you love with similar nutrition and calories. If you are trying to force down meatloaf and someone else is eating a taco, you are liable to abandon the diet for what you like.

Remake your own favorites with lower calorie sauces, spices and meat substitutions.

Find nutritional foods that you love and it will become a fitness lifestyle and not a diet.

If you love crunchiness like nuts, a bland diet will be punishment. Substitute in chia seeds and unbuttered popcorn to give your diet the crunch you desire.

This challenge is about you and what works for you as an individual. You were successful the moment you stepped on the fitness train and decided to change your life. You have the ability, through example, to impact others around you to reach their higher potential. You do not fail if your train takes a dip in the track and slows down or stops for a moment. You only fail if your train quits running its course completely and refuses to get back on track.

DAY 9

Good morning.
Yesterday we talked about finding a program that worked with your lifestyle. Each of us is uniquely different and each of us has different needs. Let's take that a step further.

You have to THINK about what food choices you are eating and how it affects you the next few hours. Most people on a diet blindly put food in their mouths according to the diet instructions without taking the time to look at how it is interacting with them. For example: Two people on the exact same diet have portions of lean meat and carbohydrates. One person may need slightly more meat than carbohydrates to keep them from being hungry and snacking until the next food break. The other person might get sleepy from that amount of protein, and need less protein and slightly more carbohydrates for energy.

Wake up folks. We are not factory copies. We are especially created to function at our own highest level. While the body will adapt to almost anything we throw at it (another miracle in itself) we hit optimal functioning when given our own combination of nutrients to match our unique lifestyle and physical needs. Some people have lifestyles that utilize more protein earlier in the day, and some people do better later in the day. It depends on how your activity level ebbs and flows.

Take the time to look at how you feel during the next hour after eating your meals today. Sometimes simply tweaking your protein or carbohydrate at a particular time of day may be what you need to reach success. And when you do, don't forget to marvel at how fearfully and wonderfully we are created.

We spend so much time mentally hating our bodies that we sometimes forget to marvel at how well it has taken our abuse, how it still manages to digest food, move oxygen, blood and nutrients around our bodies to keep our internal organs operating, and gives us the ability to move in our environments. Each one of us is a living miracle.

DAY 10

Good morning.
It may be time to reweigh yourself and check your progress. If you are excited about how well you have done with the nutrition side of things, when you get on the scale it will definitely show. If you lost some pounds...great start!

Here's the catch...those who are not exercising will show the weight go down, but so will the muscle percentage and the body fat may actually be slightly higher. You are achieving skinny fat. I don't know about you, but aside from a lower weight being healthier on the heart, organs, and joints, most of us would like to end up looking fit and trim when we are done, not saggy and out of shape. And that doesn't cover the feeling of still being tired and our bodies not being able to function at a high level.

A person can actually carry a couple of extra pounds on their bodies and as long as they are eating well they will be fairly healthy. However, our bodies are created with a multitude of muscles. If you cease to exercise you will lose more and more strength and eventually have some type of problems. That old proverb...if you don't use it, you loose it...is true when applying it to muscles.

Twenty years ago, a person could walk into a gym and start a fairly strenuous exercise program. Now that we have left the farm and factory lifestyle and become a nation that primarily sits, we find almost 80% of people come into the gym with some type of injury that they need to work around.

Usually this involves back, knee, shoulder or ankle pain. Because our bones, muscles, and joints all interconnect, when a person has a problem in one area, it will often lead to problems in other areas. And as you age and loose muscle, your physical aches and pains will start to compound.

I can't emphasize enough how important it is to get off the couch and do something. If you have to start by walking 5 minutes and resting, then that's a start. Eventually you will walk 10 minutes and then 15 and increase from there. Cardio will carry oxygen to all parts of your body. It will help carry nutrients that your body needs to heal, it will give you energy, it will help speed up your metabolism, it will help burn fat, and help your immune system.

As soon as you can add weights...do it! Weights will help build bone density, it will help you burn fat 24 hours a day, it will give you the strength to lift objects, and it will help you move through your environment without injury. It can bring your body back into alignment, and regain your shape. Muscle is one fifth the size of the same weight in fat.

That means that two people may weigh the same, but the person who is all muscle will be one fifth the size of the person who is all fat. Hmm...Skinny fat is NOT where it's at.

People have the misconception that muscle will bulk them up. That's because we watched a generation of steroid users enhance their look through drugs. The person losing weight will find that muscles help them burn calories faster, look better when they get to their goal, and be smaller and fitter than someone of the same weight who does not exercise. They will have more ability to enjoy the sports and fun times they are missing as a heavy person.

If you have been working on the nutrition part of your weight loss, now is the time to get your exercise on track. Get into the gym and ask for help getting started. Or start a walking program in your neighborhood. Or just get up and move.

We are all trying to find a path to the top of the mountain. One person will choose one path, another person will go at it another way. But when we get to the top, the view will be the same. Just make it a priority to not be the person who sits down on their journey and never makes it to the top.

DAY 11

Good morning.
 Let's talk a little about the exercise side of things. Your body will plateau after about a month. That's because we are fearfully and wonderfully designed to adapt to our surroundings and what we demand of our bodies. That means that walking program you started....the one that kicked your butt when you first started it...is no longer having the same results (heart pounding, struggle to finish), that it did when you first started.

There are many ways to take this up to the next level. Basically, if you are able to play on your cell phone, or read a book while you are exercising, then it is time to re-evaluate your program.

Your heart is a muscle...just like all your other muscles. And it needs to be pushed a bit in order to get stronger like your other muscles. The point of cardiovascular exercise is to get your heart pumping so that blood carries oxygen to all parts of your body. This will help your immune system, speed healing (sore muscles are tiny injuries you have caused while exercising), raise metabolism (that means fat burning), and raise your hormonal levels (makes you feel good, stops depression, elevates your energy). But you have to get your heart rate up to do this.

The point is to stay within your fitness level and build from there. The really great news is that you can never beat your own fitness level, so you can always progress at your own rate, while not competing against anyone else.

An example of how to do this would be to warm up and move into your normal cardio routine. If you were going for a walk, this would mean getting past that first few sluggish minutes when you are just starting and get to that slightly faster pace that you normally walk for 30 minutes. At that point you can begin doing intervals where you work REALLY HARD for 10-15 seconds then slow down to a normal pace for as long as it takes to bring your breathing down. (This might be 30 seconds or 3 minutes. It's when your body recovers.) Repeat the 10-15 seconds of hard work, followed by your recovery time.

If you are significantly overweight, your normal pace might be a shuffle and your hard work might be a strong walk. The hard work should be enough to get your heart pounding and make you feel like, "I can do this for 10-15 seconds, but I would not be able to do this for 2 minutes." It should never be to the point of making you dizzy or feel like you will pass out. Someone who is really fit might be doing a normal pace at a jog, and their 10-15 seconds would be a sprint. It's all about who you are and where you are at.

As your fitness level improves you can make the 10-15 second intervals longer, and your recovery intervals can become shorter. This type of personal training can be done on anything that raises your heart rate: Rowing machine, step machine, elliptical trainer, treadmill, walking, running, swimming, biking, etc. A smart person will alternate the types of exercise they are doing. (Even though an elliptical and treadmill both use leg muscles, they use them in slightly different ways. This makes the body have to work a bit harder to adapt to the different pressures you are putting on it. It also keeps you from being bored.)

More good news....because you are working out much harder, you can shorten that 30 minute walk, into a 20 minute body transformation. You don't have to work out longer as you plateau. You can work out shorter and smarter.

Above all, enjoy your exercise experience. That tough, "this is kicking my tush", feeling means you are alive and moving ahead with passion. You are no longer in that dead zone on the couch munching your life away in someone else's soap opera on TV. Exercise is not easy, but the results in health, wellness, and your ability to live your life, are beyond any temporary feelings of difficulty.

DAY 12

Good morning. So you've been at this challenge for a while now. Some of that first excitement and enthusiasm is starting to wear off and you have to continue the hard work. Guess what? Hard work isn't going to kill you. But layers of fat and lack of using this amazing body that you were blessed with will. You might have dropped a couple of pounds and be feeling good about yourself. That pain of how awful you looked and depressed about what you have become is not quite as strong as last week. This is NOT the time to let back your guard!

Imagine that you had a rope around your neck choking off your wind. If you couldn't get air, it would become the most important thing in your life. Survival would kick in and nothing else would matter but that next breath of oxygen. When you make healing your body and recreating this temple you live in the most important thing in your life for the next 8 weeks, you WILL be successful. That means that you might miss a little sleep to get up earlier and work out or pack your lunch. You might miss that party to get to the gym. You might have to work out on your lunch break. You will NOT use any excuse for missing a work out or eating your meals on time or making good food choices. YOU WILL BECOME A WINNER!

And guess what? The second your mind chooses to be an athlete, your body will have no choice but to change to match your minds image. Fitness is created through your thoughts, which directs your body. Your body doesn't get lazy. Your mind does. Regardless of what you look like now, when you choose to be fit at all costs, and set yourself into a consistent pattern of pushing yourself to the next level, your body will react by changing.

Be patient. Sometimes our body has to work hard to repair the damage we have done and redesign itself because you've spent a long time neglecting it. But whether you see it immediately or not, there is a miraculous work going on inside you...cells renewing, metabolism becoming higher, fat burning...that is transforming the body into the new image you hold in your head.

DAY 13

Good morning.

I heard someone refer to themselves as a gym rat. Gym rat.... Workout junkie.... What negative connotations and yet if any one of us could make it to that label we'd be well on our way to fitness success. I'll take gym rat over couch potato any day!

Part of fitness, is balancing our exercise to meet our goals. If you just do cardio, you miss tightening your body with strength training, which also builds bone density and keeps you from injury when you go about your day lifting and twisting things in your environment.

Weight lifting is not about just tightening your tush. Lean muscle uses a lot of calories to exist, in effect burning fat faster all day, even when you are at rest. More calories burned will mean a leaner you that gets to your goal at a faster rate than doing cardio alone. And because muscle is one fifth the size of the same weight in fat, you will look significantly better being 145 pounds and wearing a size 8 than you would look being a flabby 145 pounds wearing size 13.

Like cardio, there are many choices of how to lift weights. And whatever choice you make needs to be varied every month so that your body will not adapt and plateau. An easy formula is to do 3-4 sets, increasing your weight a bit and decreasing your repetitions with each set.

 For example: Your first set of about 12 is your warm-up set. It is also 'how strong am I today' set. You want to lift as much as you can (with correct form) and still be able to complete 12 repetitions. Each time you weight lift, this first set may be different as you become stronger and more able to do the work.

Each set of lifts you do will warm your body up more and help it lift the next heavier set. (Kind of like when you go for a walk and after a few minutes you will be able to walk harder and faster as your body warms up.) So for your next set you can add a few pounds of weight. This needs to be an amount that is difficult enough to just get out your next amount of reps. When you are lifting this second set of weights, you can push for about 10 repetitions. (Because you are working harder by lifting more, you can do it for a shorter amount of time.)

You can raise your weight amount again for the next set. You are working harder again so you can decrease the amount of times you lift...do about 8 repetitions.

If you choose to do a fourth set, you can raise your weight again and do about 6 repetitions.

Whichever set is the last set you perform, it needs to be done until failure. Remember that your body adapts. If you can easily do a few more repetitions it has no reason to push to change. If you are at failure, your body must change to be able to handle the pressure that it was just handed in case that pressure comes it's way again.

Don't worry about bulking up. If you are trying to lose weight, you need the extra muscle to help you get there. And as you are taking in fewer calories and will be doing a different type of workout next month, you are not going to have muscles bulging out of your body in every direction. You will look hotter in that dress or those tight jeans when you are done with your transformation. Tight ten looks way better than saggy seven.

A word of caution: Weight lifting puts tiny tears in your muscle which makes your body rush to heal and become stronger. That's why you get sore. It can take up to the 5th day before you have recovered enough to lift heavy with that body part again. So separate your lifting into parts of your body (upper body, lower body, push muscles, pull muscles, chest and biceps, etc.) then don't do weight training on that area again until about the 5th day. Do your largest body parts first. (Because it takes your arms to move the weight when doing a chest or back exercise, you may not be able to do an effective chest or back workout if you worked your arms first and they are tired).

Above all, enjoy your journey. Exercise is a tiny part of our busy day. But it has some of the greatest rewards.

DAY 14

Good morning.
Ever notice that we all seem to have a story from our
child hood that explains why we are like we are today?
Somebody didn't pay us enough attention. Someone
teased us. Someone neglected us. Somebody picked on
us. It's the reason why we don't do well in relationships.
It's why we can't lose weight. It's why we can't get ahead
in life. It's because of someone or something else that
I'm the way I am.

Because a child is completely dependent on those
around, any action that is not completely centered on
the child's happiness and needs feels like a betrayal.
That same history of stories that you've been retelling
yourself into adulthood has taken on a life of their own.
Because they are remembered as a child would see
things, they are dragged forward into the adult light of
day without an adults reasoning or filter. A child would
not see mommy coming in from a long day of work
trying to support the family and being exhausted to the
point of collapse. The child would only see mommy
being impatient and feel like they didn't match up, or
see mommy pushing them into their room and feel
neglected. A child would not see the bully living in an
angry, abusive household. A child would see daddy
yelling at him, but not realize daddy just lost his job.

Often when 'our story' is examined, in the light of
adulthood, we will lose our ability to hold the culprit
responsible. In fact, that same person can be the reason
we have had to learn to be independent, to stand up for
our self, and to achieve what we've done. It is time to
realize 'our past does not equal our future'.

No matter what has happened, we do not have to be a victim. We cannot afford to waste another moment of our lives fretting, holding grudges, looking back, and blaming someone else for our own lack of moving forward. It is truly our choice to become the best we can be. History is full of men and women who have come from terrible backgrounds and achieved great things with their lives. And graveyards are full of people who have wasted their potential and ability to be the best they can be.

You are on a challenge to transform your life. You are probably realizing that this process is as much mental as physical. We are awesome beings designed to grow and expand our knowledge. We are meant to be the best we can be in everything we do. By letting go of any negative in your past, you are making the choice to take responsibility for your own future. If you fall short, it is a simple choice to shake yourself off, recommit and get back on the track again. You have taken control of your destiny.

DAY 15

Good morning.
Look around you. How's your environment? Are you
organized and ready to go? Does your home invite you
to come in and relax, release your cares of the day,
soothe and rejuvenate your spirits, nourish your body,
and get the deep relaxing sleep you need to heal your
body of the tough workouts you are giving it?

Or do you dread going home? Do you feel out of sorts,
cluttered and irritated at home? Is your cabinets and
refrigerator filled with morsels of fat and sugar just
beckoning to you to reach for them when you are feeling
weak? It may seem silly to worry about what's around
us when we are dedicating our lives to a transformation,
but your environment is a part of you.

Transformation is about setting yourself up for success.
That includes keeping yourself mentally healthy as your
body changes. And that means making sure you
eliminate emotional eating by having a haven of serenity
and health to retreat to.

DAY 16

Good morning.
Still hanging in there and working on your fitness?
Because quitting is not an option. You tried quitting in
the past and look where that got you: Unhappy and
unhealthy. Stumbling? That happens occasionally and
we just get up and move forward again.

If you are at your dream job and have a bad day at
work, you don't quit....you just reassess what went
wrong and move on. If you are learning to play an
instrument, you can expect to hit some wrong notes.
You figure out what went wrong and keep practicing.
When you are raising your children and have a stressful
day, you don't quit being a parent... you deal with it.

Fitness works the same way. It is a part of your life and
can be viewed as necessary as brushing your teeth every
day. You choose a time...you exercise. You plan healthy
meals...you eat healthy meals. Sometimes those are
hard things to juggle. Oh well. Nobody said it would be
easy. Life often isn't. But it's necessary. You can pay the
price now or you can pay the price later in bad health,
sickness, and obesity.

I had someone ask me about a new diet on the market
that tells you what to eat and what type of exercise to do
for your body type. A few years ago it was how to diet
according to your blood type. When did Americans quit
thinking for them selves and start following the flock
like silly chickens? We are making others rich as we
race around snatching up the next pill, plan, or promise
to help us lose weight.

Folks, it is about calories in and calories out. Green coffee is a great new solution to help burn fat, but let's be real. A cork bottle of green coffee is not going to make you skinny if you keep eating two fast food meals a day and a quart of ice cream. If you get liposuction and keep eating excess calories, the weight will just show up somewhere else on your body. Take a breath. Get a grip, buckle down, and start doing the work that is necessary to transform you.

Porter Freeman once wrote a phrase he picked up somewhere. "Winning is not normal and those who constantly win follow an 'abnormal' path. The discipline, dedication and sacrifices are incomprehensible to those thousands standing outside, looking in, who are capable of joining the winning team, yet unwilling to pay the price of admission. Winners win in a fair effort, on a level playing field; because they deserve to win... they willingly pay their dues in full, time after time, after time."

DAY 17

Good morning.
When you are interacting and thinking about your
nutrition you are more conscious about what you put in
your mouth.

Remember when it used to be easy to drop a few
pounds...but now it seems impossible? There are some
things going on, as we get older, that we need to be
aware of. It's no secret that our hormonal levels go
down. Testosterone and Estrogen are not just about our
sexuality and raising kids.

A woman's body uses about 1100 calories a month to
produce that female cycle. That's good for adding a few
extra pounds every year for older women who may have
never had to worry about weight before...and for those
who are struggling...ouch!

And for men it can be a vicious cycle: Low testosterone
levels increase weight gain...and weight gain lowers
testosterone levels. Low testosterone levels lead to
insulin resistance which leads to abdominal obesity.

High intensity exercise is the way to increase hormonal
levels and help with weight loss. That 'feel good' high
you experience after intense exercise is a spike in your
hormones. It not only helps with fat burning, but
counteracts depression and speeds metabolism. It is not
a permanent situation. You must do regular, ongoing
exercise to keep the positive mental wellbeing and fat
metabolism going.

For years we have maintained that weight comes off
your body equally and you cannot spot reduce by doing
a few sit-ups: You must get your body fat down to see
your abs.

Recent studies have just come out that shows super high intensity exercise will actually target that brown belly fat that is around your abdominal area. This exercise is similar to interval training. Interval training brings your heart rate up, and then backs off for a while to let you recover. Super high intensity is done by pushing your heart rate up (never to the point of dizziness or pain), catching your breath, but not letting your heart rate come all the way down, and immediately doing another set of pushing yourself. Make sure you have a doctor's permission to do anything intense and listen to your body. If you are losing correct form or pushing yourself to a level that makes you feel faint, you may do more harm than good. Like anything else, common sense and how your body feels is your first guide.

For older folks, strength training may be safer to start with. It is low-impact compared to running, walking, or jogging. There are fewer repeating joint movements when compared to cardiovascular exercise. You can bring your heart rate up with compound movements. The progressive loading will make significant changes in body muscle versus fat percentage. This means a stronger body that will enjoy a better quality of life.

DAY 18

Good morning.

Most of us have long since realized that we can only be in one place at a time. For some reason this doesn't stop us from running around at an insane pace trying to be everything to everybody.

Sometimes we get lost in the process. When you glance at what you have to do today, take a moment to throw out anything that is unnecessary and combine tasks to simplify your day. Then make an effort to be present and fully immersed in what you do have to do.

For example: If you are doing homework with your child, don't multitask and pay bills. Let your child know he is valuable and important by giving him/her your full attention while you interact.

When you go to work...Don't drag in the local gossip and stand around wasting time. Don't text on your cell phone. Leave everything else behind and concentrate on being the best employee you can be, regardless of how others act around you.

It works the same for your fitness... When you pack your meals, take a moment to make sure you are making the healthiest choices possible. Make sure you pack enough in case your schedule changes and you can't get back home at the usual time. Make sure you aren't forgetting anything. Your nutrition is an important part of taking care of yourself.

When you exercise... Leave your cares at the door of the gym, at the start of your bike ride, or at the beginning of your walk. This is not the time to meander while you gossip with your neighbor or worry about the fight you had with your spouse. This is a small amount of time during your day, when you need to concentrate on putting in a hundred percent effort to move yourself to the next level. This is the place you are at the moment and you don't want to waste your precious time walking away no fitter than when you started.

We can remember the motto, "Just for today I will eat well, exercise hard, and live at my highest potential." All the worry and stress in the world will not give you a better quality life or help you live longer. If we make taking care of ourselves our number one priority we will have more energy and attention for our loved ones and our positive outlook will impact everything around us.

DAY 19

Good morning.
When was the last time you really noticed what a child looks like? Not saw a child...really looked at a child. Every one is different from the next, and yet they are awesomely created. They reach for something, their hands stretch out, their fingers curl around a toy. They don't think about what they are doing. Their body just responds to their needs and wants.

A child, who does not spend most of their day inside, tends to stand straight and walk tall. They bounce back and forth, full of energy, skip sideways, jump over cracks, do cart wheels, balance on curbs, walk backwards, and jump rope. The muscle, in all parts of their bodies, continually adapts to meet the needs of their lifestyles.

Our bodies are designed to move and the miracle of our blueprint is that, with the right nutrients and sleep, we can heal and even overcome obstacles like disease. Our bodies quietly and efficiently figures out a way to meet the demands we place on it.

Consider the body of a mom who is nursing. When the child needs more nutrition and consumes all of the mother's milk, the mother's body responds to this demand by creating more milk for the next feeding. How perfect is that? And as the child begins eating and needs the mother's milk supply less, the mother's body produces less milk until there is no longer a need for this source of nutrition. Again, the body adapts to the needs placed on it.

When we are seeking to improve our fitness, it is important to push ourselves to work out harder, lift heavier weights, stretch our muscles further, and do our cardio more intensely. Our body has already adapted to the poor fitness level we have. If we place demands on it by always pushing our workouts, our bodies will respond by becoming leaner, stronger, and more able to do activity. But the key is placing demands on our body. Why should your body change if you plod along at the same pace, or complete the same old workout at the same weights that you have done for the last two months? Your body does not see a need to change.

Often it is the mind that holds us back. When children are learning to walk, they fall down continually. They do not know what failure is, so they get up... and get up... and get up, until their muscles become strong enough to hold them, their balance stabilizes, and presto...they are walking. Somewhere along the way, adults have compared themselves to others and quit trying. They no longer believe in themselves.

Think of a hundred dollar bill. You may drop it in the mud, crinkle it, and even tear and tape it, but ultimately it still spends the same. It has a value of a hundred dollars. You still have the same value and ability you were created with. Somewhere you stopped believing in your value. Your body doesn't know this. It just does what you demand it to do, which can often be nothing but sitting on the couch watching TV.

As soon as you remove that mountain of disbelief that you have rising in front of you, and demand your body to take action, it will adapt to the occasion and work to meet that demand. You may have to fall and get up...and get up...and get up, as your body gets stronger and your balance and flexibility increases. Ultimately the vision you hold in your head, is the vision you will become. Failure is NOT an option!

DAY 20

Good morning.
One area that is most confusing to people, is nutrient timing. The people, who benefit most from WHEN you take in your nutrients along with WHAT and HOW MUCH, is your athletes and people who are struggling to lose weight.

Any nutrition program that has a person taking in fewer calories than they utilize will result in weight loss. How deprived and hungry a person feels, whether their body has enough energy to feel good, and if their nutrition is optimal to build lean muscle, can be helped with timing and food choices.

THE BASICS: If you have the ability to choose whole food (preferably unprocessed) on your nutrition plan, your body will be more satisfied and adapt more naturally to a lifestyle change that you can maintain, and not feel like you are dieting. For instance... you can drink a shake that has 800 calories in it and feel extremely full...for a while. Because it goes into your body quickly, your body does not register the amount of calories, but rather does a quick digestion and looks for the next meal. You will soon be looking for something to munch on. If you ate a full 800 calorie meat and vegetable dinner, your body will experience the entire chewing/digestion process and be satisfied for a much longer time.

If you break your meals and snacks into smaller time frames about 2-3 hours apart, your body will maintain a more stable blood sugar (think stable energy), and both digestion and calorie burning will become more efficient. This means eliminating the low blood sugar search for munchies, and your body using more total daily calories to digest meals and snacks multiple times. If two people ate the exact same thing, the person who separated their meals into more frequent meals will be more successful in losing weight and have a higher metabolism than the person who just eats a few times a day.

Balance your meals with proteins and carbohydrates. This may be slightly different for each person. Again we remind you to THINK about how you feel the hour after you eat. If you are sleepy, you may need a tad less protein and a tad more carbs to keep you going. (Protein helps keep you satisfied and carbs are the gas in your tank that gives you get up and go). If you are getting hungry too quickly, add a bit more protein to that time of day.

Drink water continually all day long. Be aware that if you are drinking non calories beverages, they can trigger sugar cravings. If possible drink straight water. One way to get the caffeine without drinking a soda would be to take a green tea or type of caffeine pill.

BEFORE WORKING OUT: This meal or snack should be about an hour before doing exercise. It should be a mixture of carbs and protein, with the balance leaning heavier on the carb side for energy. It should also be low in fat and fiber so that it is easy to digest. (You don't want a chunk of meat or anything heavy in your gut when you are exercising hard). Examples might include low-fat/low sugar yogurt or milk and a banana or a natural homemade protein/carb drink.

DURING WORK OUT: Replenish with continual water consumption. You really do not need anything else unless you will be exercising for a prolonged period of time, or have not given your body adequate nutrition before your work out to maintain intensity. A vitamin enhanced beverage with or without a small amount of protein and carbs can help if you feel light headed or weak.

AFTER WORKING OUT: This meal/snack should also be a combination of protein and carbs and taken as soon as possible after working out. The purpose of this meal is to STOP protein breakdown, START Protein resynthesizing, and REPLENISH glycogen stores. The amount of calories in this meal will be dependent on your nutritional needs and goals. It can be small or larger, but needs to be easy for your body to absorb...a bit of protein bar, balanced protein drink, or some milk. If you choose to make this a snack, instead of a meal replacement, you will want to follow up with a meal in the next hour. This meal can be a heavier balance, such as a tuna and whole grain sandwich, or meat and veggies.

DAY 21

Good morning.
Ever notice how adult children seem to have the same mannerisms as their parents? Children inherit much more than eyes or a smile from their family line. They inherit values, genes (bad and good), and attitudes. It is documented that families, who deal in criminal behavior, will have a higher amount of descendants, down the line, who will be in trouble with the law. Families who value education will turn out a higher percentage of descendants who are doctors, lawyers, politicians, and business persons. Alcoholics will have a higher incidence of alcoholics in their family line, depressed people will leave a legacy of depression, and a person with an eating disorder can pass it to their kid, who passes it to their kid, who passes it to the grand kid. People who deal with the world in anger or who mistreat their families, pass these lessons on to their kids who repeat the process in their lives.

While we may be prone to these actions, we don't have to follow them. We can break the chain of addictions and behaviors that bring us down by asserting our free will...our personal choice. Your creator has placed a spiritual force in you which is greater than the forces outside of you. We were meant to achieve, not crawl on our bellies in defeat.

Look at the community around you. The world is filled with families who make poor choices in both their nutrition and exercise. They raise children who follow in their footsteps, who raise children who follow in their footsteps. It is a small wonder that obesity is considered an epidemic. Hundreds of descendants can follow in the nutritional train wreck of one set of parents.

Likewise, parents who teach and model good nutrition, and the importance and enjoyment of consistent exercise, produce a line of descendants who tend to value their bodies and take care of them. This can eliminate years of degenerative diseases brought on or aggravated by obesity.

Isn't it time to quit making excuses and take responsibility about what you are creating? You may be doing really well with your program. You may have fallen a few times. Big deal. You are a continually evolving human. At this time next year you will either be fitter or fatter. The next time you look in the face of your child or grandchild, take an opportunity to recognize characteristics that you have put there. Are they happy, healthy, optimistic, have good values and contribute in a valuable way to the community? You have the opportunity to break the cycle in your family. You have the opportunity to change the destiny of those following in your footsteps. How powerful is that?

DAY 22

Good morning.
Sometimes we are so busy telling ourselves what we did
wrong, that we forget to look at what we are doing right.
You may not have done things perfectly, but are you
sleeping better and having more energy during the day?
Have you cut down the amount of time you spend going
through fast food restaurants? Are you more aware of
what's going into your mouth? Are your clothes fitting
just a tad better? Have you exercised more and harder
this last month than you did in previous months? Are
you drinking more water these days and less sugary
beverages?

Remember that the longest journey starts with one
small step. And if you keep going, step by step, you will
eventually get to your goal. It's all about progress not
perfection. We should never compare ourselves to
anyone else because we are all walking a path that
nobody else can. Some people have run into obstacles
like work, or illness, or even worse. Some people have
run into events like weddings or birthdays or
graduations that involve yummy temptations. Some
people have run into obstacles such as their own habits,
addictions, and attitudes.

Nobody is immune from life. But you are here. You keep
coming back and continuing your journey toward fitness
and health. That alone is something awesome that you
are doing right for yourself. Use the strength of the
things you are doing right to build on and recreate
yourself. Tweak the problem areas and take things to
the next level. You may not be sailing through this
challenge. You may be clawing and dragging yourself
forward each time you fall back. But you are worth
every bit of sweat and tears you are putting into this
journey. Because when fitness becomes a lifestyle and
you are reaping your rewards of health and energy, the
taste of victory is going to be that much sweeter.

DAY 23

Good morning.
Did you sleep well? Most Americans are up long hours.
Their sleep is interrupted by cell phone messages, kids
and animals, worries, and lack of planning.

When you sleep, your brain goes through four different
cycles called Rapid Eye Movement Stages (REM). EEG
brain wave readers can tell that the brain works
differently in these stages. During the first stage, your
body relaxes and heart rate slows. Sometimes you have
a feeling of falling. During the next two stages, your
body is in a deep restful state. This is where healing and
maintenance occurs. While you rest peacefully, the
mind and body works hard to repair chemical
imbalances, heal injuries, reset blood sugar levels, and
maintain optimal brain function.

When you exercise hard, you create small tears in your
muscles that require healing. That's why you are sore. If
your body does not go through enough REM stages, it
cannot fully heal itself and you will find yourself
dragging the next day.

Lack of sleep also ages you, weakens your immune
system, effects your blood sugar and chemical balance,
raises cortisol (which effects obesity, can cause
hypertension and memory loss), reduces energy,
diminishes mood and concentration, and magnifies pain
levels. People who are sleep deprived often reach for
caffeine and sugar to counter balance their lack or
energy and, in general, eat more snacks and meals
because they are up for a longer amount of time.

Our bodies are regulated by an internal clock that resets itself every 24 hours based on night and day. Once we invented the light bulb, and increased our ability to be awake at any hour, we started to interfere with this natural rhythm. Every time we turn on a light we interrupt our Circadiun Rhythum a bit, which interrupts our bodies ability to produce proteins and chemicals at the right times. Our body is forced to work much harder. When the body is forced to work harder and longer it has trouble restoring itself.

When we are looking at being at our optimum fitness, it makes sense to plan your sleep time as carefully as you plan your meals and exercise. Your body needs a dark, sleep inducing environment that can be uninterrupted for 8-9 hours each day.

Ideally you will want to take your multiple vitamins and a bit of protein before bedtime to ensure your body has the necessary building blocks available for healing and repair. This is about building the best you. If you were building a bridge, you would not be able to complete the job without enough cement. While your body is sleeping it must have enough protein and nutrients to do the repair job required to have you at your peak performance level.

DAY 24

Good morning.
We are taught to give our time and energy to everyone
else. It seems selfish to take the time to precook and
package meals and get in our exercise. As a nation we
are just too busy. Our days are packed from wake-up to
sleep with activities.

And yet, as we gain weight, we are angry and frustrated.
We become overwhelmed by how we feel, how we look,
our lack of self-esteem, how tired we are, how depressed
we are. Isn't this pity party the completely self-involved
situation we wanted to avoid?

Now just the opposite is happening. As you schedule
your workouts and plan your meals, you have MORE
energy for family. You feel better and are a nicer person
to be around. You are starting to look up and out at life,
instead of inward.

You are a vibrant part of your community. As your self-
esteem and quality of life expands, you can reach out
and touch others. Grabbing some caffeine? Bring some
back for your co-worker. Going to Costco? Offer to pick
something up for the neighbor. Know someone who is
struggling? Pay their heating bill. Know someone with
kids? Babysit for a night and let them get out. Take
someone a basket of fruit. Drop someone a note. Give
someone a hug. Tell someone they are doing a good job.
Listen to someone (without offering your opinion).

The healthier and fitter you become, the more you can
reach out and help someone else. You can lead by
example, not nagging. And like every circle of life, the
more you bless others, the more you will feel blessed.

DAY 25

Good morning.
The amazing thing about the human mind is that it works like a powerful computer. We've talked about what comes out of your mouth will create your reality. Even if you are in the grips of an addiction you can repeat to yourself, "Food (or alcohol, or cigarettes, etc.) has no power over me. I am getting healthier every day." The power of your mind can cure you of your addiction. But you have to speak out loud, continually, to reprogram your thoughts and actions.

Your mind can not only recreate you, it can keep you moving forward. Because it is a problem solver, you only need to access your thoughts by asking the right question. "What can I eat today that will be yummier than any other option that could tempt me and still be on my nutritional program? Where, in my schedule, can I fit in a great workout today? What type of exercise can I do today to make me feel great and challenge me to the next level? What is a fun thing I could do with my family that would be fit and healthy? What can I do today to make me feel like I'm living my life with passion and reaching my potential? Who can I influence with my good example and what do I need to do in my own life to inspire that person? What's a great way to get my water in today?

The beauty of the mind is that when you ask the right questions, it immediately sets about giving you some answers. Instead of saying, "I feel out of energy today," you could say, "What can I do that will give me more energy today?" Such a simple changing of the words can unlock the power of your mind.

DAY 26

Good morning.

Everywhere you turn there is a different pill to help you lose weight. And let's face it; America has proven itself to be the first to reach for the latest gimmick that promises a shortcut to all our dreams coming true. No amount of supplements is going to make you lean and toned or buff and ripped if you are eating a carton of cookies every day. There are products that can go along with your goals to enhance the hard work you are doing.

One of the most important is a multiple vitamin. Try to get the most natural, complete source you can afford. It is almost impossible to get all the nutrition we need in our food because most of us live in an 'on the run' environment, not a 'grow your own food' environment. When you are exercising, you are often causing little tiny muscle tears. So your body is in a continual state of healing. You must have all the vitamins, minerals, and protein, your body needs, to fully recover.

When you put several supplements together, it is called a stack. Many diet pills are a combination of supplements. The choice of what you are looking for depends on your goals. Supplements can be broken down into several categories:

Fat burners that are thermogenic, giving energy and raising metabolism: Caffeine, Green Tea Extract, Citrus Aurantium/Synephrine, Yerba Mate.

Fat burners that are stimulant free: CLA, Decaffeinated Green Tea, Garcinia Cambogia, Green Coffee Bean Extract, Raspberry Ketones, Satiereal Saffron Extract, Ashwagandha, Chromium, 7-Keto.

Appetite curbs: Glucomannan Fiber

Carb and Fat Inhibitors: Chitosan, White Kidney Bean Extract, Cissus Quadrangularis.

If you choose to buy supplements, beware of mixing several together. If you take several products all containing thermogenic stimulants, you risk feeling jittery. If you cannot find a diet aid you like, you can build your own stack. However, be careful and pay attention to how your body feels and reacts. And remember, that nothing is going to do the job for you. Calories in/Calories out. Eat right/ Exercise hard/Get your sleep.

DAY 27

Good morning.

Do you have something you've done that you feel embarrassed about? Something that you won't tell anyone else about because they might judge you? Guess what? We all do! As much as we say we are an individual, there are things that we've all done that we are afraid to admit or tell others because we are terrified that we will no longer be liked or accepted. Things that are pushed deep down and hidden gnaw at us and manifest in bad health. We can't believe we can achieve great things because secretly we KNOW we are a bad person. And it effects how we treat others. A liar will suspect others of lying. A cheat will always think someone else is cheating. A thief will not trust others.

One of the hardest things we can do is take the time to actively think about those things that bring us guilt and write them down. Take the time to realize how they have impacted your life and relegate them to the past. Who or what you've done in the past does not equal the future. It's your choice to be the person you want to be going forward. You are done with that type of behavior. Burn your written paper of remorse and move on in freedom to be what you want to be. If you need to make amends for wrong you've done to someone, than get it over with. Make a choice to be free from the chains of shame that have been holding you back.

If you take the time to recognize the behavior that bothers you each week, you will soon find that little things like leaving a mess for someone else to clean up will make you uncomfortable. Your conscience will not stimulate you to over eat in an attempt to make you feel better. You are building character. And in the end you will be able to treat others better, treat yourself better, and live your best life.

DAY 28

Good morning.

Have you heard the expression, "We are made in the image of our creator?" Think about that. We are all individual and unique, so what do we have that mimics our creator? A spirit of unlimited power. It is that unique force in us that defies our body's limits. It is that deep down grit that gets a person out of his wheelchair and walking again, when the doctor says it will never happen. It's that fight to protect your family against all odds. It's that will to survive and beat a disease that is supposed to put you down. It's that human quality that comes out when the going gets tough.

Don't allow yourself to slump through life feeling beaten and flawed. You are an image of your creator. You have a power inside like no other, meant to rise and excel. You haven't seen your best day yet. It is still coming. You haven't reached your highest goal yet. You have the power to transform yourself and walk in the image you were designed to look like, and follow the path you were meant to travel. You have untold blessings waiting to be heaped on you, if you'll just pull your head out of the sand and raise up to receive them.

Don't allow anyone else's opinion, or comments to bring you down. You have been given a temple and the responsibility to take care of it. You live in this temple twenty four hours a day. If you take responsibility for this blessing, you can rise to receive even more blessings.

Too many of us wallow through life taking the easy way out. Use that infinite power you have to take control of yourself and rise to the next level. It may be tough, it may take a while, but no one can take away the power you possess to transform yourself. You can only lose your power by giving it away.

You give it away each time you choose to miss a workout, grab something unhealthy, or quit believing in yourself. You are cheating yourself of reaching your highest dreams. Put your head up, square your shoulders, pull in your gut and be proud. Recommit to taking care of yourself and being thankful for what we have been given.

Day 29

Good morning.
Heard about Creatine and wondering if it's for you?
Creatine is one of the most studied substances in the
world of exercise. It is a fairly safe amino acid that is
used to enhance performance.

Creatine works by taking more water into your cells
which helps with protein synthesis. It should be taken
just before exercising to enhance energy and your ability
to do hard work. When used in weight lifting and
explosive type exercise, it helps the user do harder,
more intense workouts, which increases muscle fiber.
The catch is to use it before exercise. If you are taking it,
but not hitting the gym, you will be gaining water weight
for no reason. And there is not a big improvement for
those doing more sedentary exercise that doesn't push
you to your limits.

Both men and women can see improvement with
Creatine use. Increase in muscle fiber means some
weight gain. With the additon of male testosterone, this
can lead to bigger, stronger muscles. With women it can
also lead to a bit of weight gain in additional muscle
building. But remember, muscle weighs significantly
more than fat. It is also much tighter and leaner.

This is a win/win for most women who want to be fit
and struggle to add a bit of muscle. Muscle looks lean
and doesn't jiggle. It lifts the booty and counteracts
gravity. Metabolically, it uses much more calories to
exist, which allows you lose weight faster and maintain
your weight better. It also gives you the strength to do
the fun things you want to do, in your life, which is
active.

When using Creatine, you should know within a week if it works for you. Pay attention to your workouts. If you are able to do more intense workouts, it is benefiting you. If your workouts seem about the same, then don't bother. Not everything works for everybody.

There have been a few (very few) questions about whether it affects your kidneys. The studies were done on people who could have been taking many other vitamins and supplements also. For the most part, studies have proved it to be completely safe, but if you have a compromised kidney, it just makes good sense to not add to the overload. People who consume lots of beef and herring will see fewer results than people who eat more carbs and vegetables. That's because there is natural Creatine in the meat sources.

Whether you use Creatine or not, you will see results from the gym if you DO THE WORK. Gyms are filled with people who jump on the treadmill and read a book or talk on their cell phones. Then they complain that their body never changes and they aren't seeing results. You have to THINK about your exercise. How can you continually change it up to keep your body working hard and come at your muscles from a different direction?

DAY 30

Good morning.
Here we are again. Are we tired of hearing the same old
stuff? "Get moving. You can do it." Sorry. There is no
magic pill invented since yesterday that is going to do
this for you. You may not be a professional at anything
else in your life, but learn to be a professional at getting
your tired butt out of the couch and do your exercise.

You may not have the highest paycheck on the block
but you can have the tightest abdominals. Sometimes
you have to quit thinking about it, and just do it. "I
should try to exercise today," is just a matter of getting
up, grabbing your sweats, and getting on with doing it.
Your body will thank you, your mind will thank you,
your self- esteem will thank you, and your energy level
will thank you. The only one who will want to thank you
while you sit on that couch, is the manufacturer who
created those potato chips or that candy.

DAY 31

Good morning.
Ever feel like today is your day. You are going to eat right. You are going to exercise. You are going to get it right today.

Then you run late at work. You forgot to grab something for dinner. Your kid needs to be run somewhere. It's getting later and later, and finally you just don't have the time or energy to workout.

Time is one of the key problems people have when faced with an exercise program. Yet exercise is one of the things that gives you the energy to have that great day. Think about getting up a bit earlier and starting your day with exercise. At first it may seem almost impossible to roll out of bed any earlier. But if you can get your body in the habit of exercising you will not only have more energy to function, but it will be out of the way. No matter what happens later, you've got it done. This means feeling better about yourself all day, taking another step toward your goals, and setting yourself up mentally to eat better and cope better so that you don't backslide.

A fitness lifestyle is all about having a good plan. Being dedicated to exercising before you do anything else reinforces that this is an important part of making fitness happen.

Here is where you can grab a supplement to help you get started. A bit of caffeine may be all you need on the way to the gym or before you head out the door to get you going. The other part of this is turning off your mind. Know you will be working out the night before. Set out your clothes so there is no chance of fumbling. When that alarm goes off, JUMP out of bed and MOVE. Don't think about how tired you are. Don't think "I could sleep an extra half hour and do this tonight". Don't allow your mind to go anywhere except "I can do a level 10 workout and change my body today!" Have that image, of what you are headed toward, firmly in your mind. Hit the floor running and GO, GO, GO!

DAY 32

Good morning.
When you are hitting close to the half way mark in your personal challenge, it is easy to be discouraged. The first momentum is wearing off, it seems like you haven't achieved as much as you thought you would. This is a critical time of your journey.

This is where some people are feeling a bit better about themselves and have lost that first painful, emotional drive that put them on the fitness path. They began to get a bit lax and the first thing they know, they've gained their weight back.

Other people have slipped so many times, they feel they haven't made any advances. They just quit trying.

Stop the spiral now. You have spent the last month learning a lot about yourself. You know what trips you up, and what has derailed you. Look at your goals, adjust them, and get moving forward.

Remember that everyone else is struggling also. Many of them are giving up. Sometimes the successful person is the one who grits their teeth and forges ahead. If you tighten up your program and make sure you are planning and packing those meals, you will find out your slip ups will become less frequent. If you continue exercising you will find that one day you will wake up and start seeing a difference.

Each day compounds on the next. History shows us that sometimes the one who does it best, that changes their destiny, which makes the biggest impact, is the one who also makes the most mistakes. The only difference is the winner is also the one who doesn't give up. They get in the game of life, and start kicking butt, again and again, no matter how many times they fall.

DAY 33

Good morning.
Most people, who struggle with fitness, feel as if there is an angel on one shoulder and a devil on the other. One part of them is saying, "Be good. Don't eat that cake. There's a lettuce leaf over there that you should eat!" The other voice in them says, "Go on. There's Sally Lou over there having a piece of cake and she's thin! One piece won't hurt."

The reality is that food is not the enemy. People who diet continually have trained their minds to constantly fight themselves. If you break your diet, you think, "I'll start again tomorrow." In the meantime you eat everything in sight because you'll be depriving yourself tomorrow. Or, if you overeat at one meal, you decide to cut your calories for the rest of the day and end up getting too hungry later. Then you binge.

We have become so concerned with our food, that we lose the ability to enjoy it. Every bite of something we truly like becomes a labor of guilt. In our heads, diet means restriction, loss of enjoyment, the ongoing punishment that is the only way to look good. And if we find a food that we really like and feel it is 'authorized' on our diet, we often feel out of control and binge on it.

When we change our mindset, food no longer controls us. If you are saving to buy a house, and your last pair of jeans had a hole in them or you ran out of shampoo, you would probably splurge and get the few things you didn't budget for. Then you'd get back on track with continuing to save.

When life comes along and someone has a birthday, having a tiny piece of cake to celebrate should not be a license to finish your day in a full out binge. It's about balance. If you are exercising consistently and packing meals ahead of time, you take out the need to obsess about every mouthful. Special events should not derail your journey... they should be a guilt free time of sharing with others.

Fitness is about lifestyle. It's not about a diet. It's time to kick the angel and devil off your shoulder and get real.

DAY 34

Good morning.
Emotional eating is a reaction to our environment. Like
any addiction, we get something from it. When you are
stressed, in an argument, overworked, overtired, lonely,
have bad self-esteem, are depressed, are frightened or
hopeless, you are in a state of pain. At that point your
life is so overwhelming that you need to escape. The
feelings, during the moment you are in, are bigger than
the need to stop the addiction... and the addiction offers
the relief you need to get through the moment.

Eating temporarily distracts the mind, gives you that
temporary emotional buffer, gives you temporary energy,
and a temporary feeling of enjoyment. We all know that
'temporary' goes away and we now have the additional
burden of guilt, disgust, and self-hate going on. But
there is our addiction, beckoning gently, to distract us
from our pain again.

It is easier to break a habit when you substitute another
habit in its place. It is one thing to say, "I'm going to
paint my nails or go for a walk when I feel like
overeating", but that plan is not too effective when you
are in the middle of a busy work day and your boss is
snarling at you, or your child has the flu and has
projectile pooped and vomited on you for three days and
you've only been able to sleep three hours. You will not
be painting your nails at that moment, but that tray of
donuts sitting on the counter, or that drive through
window on your break, takes the pressure off just fine.

Our body is a creature of habit. We will go through a pattern of thought and actions when we reach for our addiction. For instance: Somebody does something that you feel upsets you. You become defiant and angry. Your body reacts by being tense and rigid. Your mind works you into a state of self- righteousness and you tell yourself you DON"T CARE about the diet...you are just going to eat. And you do...lots. The food helps to buffer the angry feelings, tastes good, and gives you some temporary energy to go with that anger and get something done. Eventually, when the anger goes away, you have now eaten 5000 calories and feel depressed and weepy.

You may be depressed. Your self talk tells you all the reasons life is worthless and you are worthless. Your body mimics this by the way it slumps and your mouth turns down. What ever. You don't care. You will never get it right. You will never get this weight off. You will never get past your problems. It's hopeless. It doesn't matter if you pick up that donut...and another...and another. Again you have a buffer...it's yummy...it distracts your thoughts...it gives you some temporary energy...and you are feeling fine. Eventually, the feeling goes away, you have now eaten 5000 calories and the depression starts all over.

When you are breaking an addictive habit like eating, you have to choose a replacement habit that works with your lifestyle. It has to be accessible immediately, and it has to be able to distract your mind as quickly and completely as food does. It is important to realize your own patterns. What are you thinking when you are building toward a binge? What do you do with your body posture that reflects those thoughts? If you know your pattern, you can substitute the new pattern of habit when the old one begins to take place before it is too late to stop.

Choosing something that uses your other senses can be super powerful. Identify some time in your life when you felt extremely happy and serene. (Right after the birth of a child, a loving moment with someone special, your wedding, etc).

Meditate on these happy thoughts each day for a week or so, until you FEEL the happy scene easily when you think about that event. Find a scent that reminds you of that event. (A baby lotion that makes you think of the birth, the cologne of that special person, the pine scent of the tree during that special Christmas, etc.) When you smell that scent, you want to immediately feel like smiling, sitting up straight, and feeling relaxed and radiant.

Find a picture that takes you to that special event: Picture of your child, a special vacation, your new house, etc. Put this picture on your desk. Put it on your refrigerator. Hang it on your mirror. Put it on your TV..

Find an object that relates to your special time. (A soft piece of flannel that feels like a baby blanket, a plastic flower that looks like a flower you were given at a special moment, a piece of ribbon in the color you wore to your graduation, etc.)

Find some music that makes you feel powerful, happy, relaxed, or content.

Use your toolbox of senses; smell, sight, hearing and touch, to bring you into a state of power, serenity, and happiness when you recognize your body moving toward an addictive state.

When your boss is standing over you snarling, you can reach into your pocket and touch your item that brings you feelings of joy. You can glance at your picture that brings you happiness and consciously relax and let the snarling flow over you.

When you are late and fighting traffic, you can think about your special moment and let your body relax. You can breathe in the scent that takes you to a happy time through a hanky or item you have put scent on. You can glace at the picture on your dashboard of the place you love and find calmness.

If you are somewhere alone, you can close your eyes and meditate on that time that brings a smile to your face. You can feel the feelings you felt then. You can choose the happy state you are in.

If you are home feeling depressed, you can put on that music that takes you into a happy state, and you can look at the pictures that make your life serene. You can throw a scent into the water on the stove and recreate happy memories.

The power of recreating good habits is choosing something that can change your state of mind immediately and with the same effectiveness as the habit you are breaking. With practice, the body will reach for the new habit. The feelings of success and control you achieve each time you avoid the old addictive behavior will fuel the use of the new habit. Like anything, it takes practice, practice, practice.

Day 35

Good morning.
Have you noticed that most things we strive for takes time? A person will dedicate themselves to 2-4 years of college to get a degree that may or may not get them a job. We equate a longer amount of time to reach our goal to a greater reward.

And yet, after years of abuse to our bodies, when we decide to lose weight we want to do it...NOW! We look for that miracle cure to take twenty pounds off this month...preferably without eating right or exercising. And if we are doing the work to get the results, we want it to be quicker, easier, and without taking time from the rest of our activities. What an irrational way of thinking when everything else about our world is a process.

If you approached your weight loss as you would deciding to go back to school, you would be happier, more prepared and more successful. To get a degree, you have to know the goal you are going for. You have to commit to giving up time and activities, in other areas of your life, to do the work it takes to succeed. You have to have a clear understanding that you will be at this, as long as it takes, until you reach your goal...it is not a ten minute process. It is a plan for your life that will impact how you live and how you end up. When you settle down, and commit to doing this for the duration, even if it takes 2-4 years, you will be prepared to weather life's up and downs and stay committed to the final goal.

Stop the insanity of trying to squish your long term goal, of being fit and losing weight, into the short term, "I want to look good for this event," timeline. Those who love and know you won't love you any less if you are twenty pounds heavier than you wanted to be at the event. And you won't be raising your stress level, pushing your body into a fad diet, and packing the twenty pounds back on after the event. Take your time. Do it right. Make fitness part of your every 'school' day. Your body will love you. Your family will love the calmer, happier you. And the weight will stay off.

DAY 36

Good morning.

People often overlook the importance of water when they are seeking that magic pill to lose weight. We have discussed the body's ability to adapt to whatever you give it, or don't give it, in this case. Water helps metabolize stored fat.

Your liver works on metabolizing fat into useful energy. When you don't give your body enough water, the kidney can't flush effectively and so the liver has to help the kidneys. This results in less metabolized fat... more fat remains in the body, and weight loss stops.

When your body feels threatened by lack of water, it reacts by retaining water. This water is stored in the body (legs, feet, etc.) The way to get rid of the excess is to drink more water. This puts the body at optimum fluid levels and it allows the retained fluid to leave.

When you are overweight, you need more water than a thin person...about a glass for each additional 25 pounds. And the body needs a steady intake, of 8-12 glasses daily, to be at proper fluid level. (8 to maintain basic fluid levels and up to 12 to properly hydrate skin). Fluid levels may also need to be increased if the weather is hot or if you exercise more.

So here is the bonus...If you can get your water levels to optimum levels, hunger disappears. Your body hums along doing its job of metabolizing fat and flushing the extra waste out of the body that is produced through weight loss. Your muscles can maintain proper tone. Your cells are flushed and healthy which helps the cell shrinkage and keeps your skin resilient. This in turn helps to eliminate that saggy skin that is left when you lose weight.

To maximize the effectiveness of water, try to drink it cold which has a bit of a metabolism effect as the body has to heat the water.

- Drink 2 glasses of water after waking up to get your internal organs activated.
  * Drink 1 glass 30 minutes before each meal (but not closer, because you do not want to dilute stomach acid which is needed to digest food.)
  *Drink 1 glass of water before a bath or shower to help lower blood pressure.
  * Drink 1 glass of water before bed to help reduce the risk of heart attack or stroke.

By drinking water consistently through the day, you help reduce the risk of flushing too many nutrients which will cause a water intoxication effect. And your body stays at peak fluid levels. Try to put a good quality water filter on your sink at home, or add some good tasting powdered vitamin C to your chlorinated tap to neutralize the chlorine.

DAY 37

Good morning.

Let's face it. You have to be mentally tough to lose weight. Every day in America you will run into temptations and food that can easily derail your nutrition plan. After all, a drug addict can just quit the drug. You still have to eat...right? It's much harder to break a food habit.

Or is it? No one stuffed that double cheeseburger and fries down your throat. Nobody held a gun to your head and forced you to eat half a chocolate cake and four candy bars. Get real. You are the reason you are fat and out of shape. It was you who chooses to sleep in instead of getting out of bed a half hour early to exercise. It is not your body that hasn't had the strength to lose weight...it's your mind.

By the time 4-6 weeks have gone by in a weight loss program almost everyone will have fallen off the wagon, and many will stop trying completely. So if you've slipped up...have you failed? Of course not! If Albert Einstein or Bill Gates gave up when they failed, we would be back at the starting gate.

Let's get back to work. Did you write out your goals when you started this journey? Don't whine about how hard it is to lose weight if you haven't even made your goal important enough to write down, along with a plan of how to get there.

When you have your goal and plan to get there, write down what it will feel and look like if you make it to your goal. How will your life change and what can you accomplish toward your dreams?

Write down what your life will be like and how you will feel and what dreams will wither and die if you give up. When you look back from your death bed, will you feel you lived your life with passion or will you regret the wasted time?

Two things motivate us in life: Pleasure and Pain. Pain is the bigger motivator. We will procrastinate about doing something because the reward of getting it done is less than the discomfort of doing it. But when the pain becomes great enough we will finally get it done. Make your list of what you are losing out on, in your unfit lifestyle, very clear. This is your motivation to keep moving.

When you break your diet, the pleasure of the cookie is closer than the pain that follows later. It is important to keep the picture of what we will feel and look like in front of you so that the pain of failure is stronger than the temporary urge to give in.

Now take your goals, short and long term, and read them out loud daily. Visualize about how you will act and feel when you reach your goal. Practice visualizing how you should react when faced with a tempting situation. Know ahead of time what you will say and do when faced with a treat you weren't prepared to be around. Think of a person who is fit that you would love to be like, and ask yourself what they would do in that situation. Meditation and visualization is your key to mental success. That and a positive attitude that says, "I WILL NOT GIVE UP! I WILL BE SUCCESSFUL!" You want to win the weight loss game? Quit making excuses and do your homework.

DAY 38

Good morning.
So if you have been struggling, I assume you have now gone back, rewritten your goals and figured out what is motivating you to keep going and what the pain is if you don't keep going. Did you put these on a card to carry around with you? Did you pack your meals for the day, and do you have your items, that use your other senses, to distract yourself.

Have you taken a few moments to visualize where you are going and meditate on success?

Are you starting your day with 2 glasses of water? And pushing that water all day? Remember, your fluid levels have to be adequate in your body to suppress your appetite. It's not the actual glass of water that fills you, because that feeling of fullness will go away in a short while. It's the overall hydration of the body, that sends the signal, which tells your body it can quit craving.

Have you brought your 'get it done' attitude? You choose your mindset, not the situations around you. Are you determined and strong minded enough to stick with your plan, even if everything else seems to be falling apart? Because the reality is, the most successful people in the world have stress and life situations also. The only thing that separates them from you is the mindset. And you have the same ability, the same awesome potential to transform yourself. Fight for yourself and your happiness.

DAY 39

Good morning.
Did you wake up thankful today? Or did you avoid your mirror or mentally throw up your hands when you saw your reflection? Are you thankful for your body?

That military vet who came back without legs would tell you to be thankful for legs that will carry you across the room. That multiple Sclerosis patient will tell you to be grateful for the muscles that support your activities...because theirs won't. That cancer victim will tell you to be thankful for the energy you have to get on with your life. The person with asthma will tell you to be thankful for the breaths you breathe and not take them for granted. That Alzheimer patient would tell you to be thankful for your mind...if they could remember what their mind is for. That person who is abused might tell you to be thankful for your spirit of kindness, because not everyone has one. Everywhere you go there is someone who would be thankful for what you've got, even if it is not as perfect as you'd like it.

It's time to put things in perspective. Your body, your spirit, your mind is valuable and precious. You need to take care of it. You have so much to offer, that someone else may not have. You are a work in progress, and just because that work is not finished, does not mean you can't be thankful for where you're at. Your journey and struggles will give you the compassion to reach out to someone else in a similar situation. Your friends and loved ones will not quit loving you if haven't attained your goal yet.

Remember your value and be thankful. Have the calmness of spirit to be happy with where you are at and where you are going. You have been created with the tools to get there.

DAY 40

Good morning.
When was the last time you rewarded yourself (other than eating)? When we are depressed or angry we reach for something sweet or fatty to make us feel good. That is a reward. Rewards can be just as motivating when used for weight loss.

Consciously choose things that you enjoy to use as motivation. For instance..."I'll take time to do my nails tonight if I stay on track with my nutrition today." Small things that you think you'd like to have or do in advance for moving yourself in a positive way.

Small daily rewards can be taking the time to make a small meatloaf or something healthy you love for dinner. Or choose something that doesn't involve food: Stickers or smiley faces to go on your calendar on your successful days, a night of music or dancing, a bubble bath, a massage and/or favorite TV show, a foot rub, a scalp rub.

Things you could do for a weekly non-gain or weight loss...A favorite magazine, shower gel or cologne, a new make-up product, lip gloss or body lotion, a healthy meal out, a movie, a dance class or event, a bike ride, a professional facial or massage, a haircut or color, a card party, a new clothing piece or jewelry.

As you lose larger amounts of weight along the way, you could treat yourself to a weekend away, an outfit, a spoil yourself spa weekend, an mp3 player or heart rate monitor, new exercise shoes, or just new shoes, or a makeover.

Be creative and stay within your budget. But plan your treats to match your goals and interests. You will find the money you save from eating at fast food joints and binging on sweets will give you a few more dollars that you can use as reward money. And remember...if you are only getting treats when you are emotional and reaching for food, what message are you sending your body and mind? A consistent reward program can motivate you to move forward and allow you to smell the roses as your travel down your weight loss path.

DAY 41

Good morning.

Relax. You can only be in one place at a time. You are right where you are supposed to be in your journey. If you haven't made it to where you thought you would be in your fitness and weight loss...that's OK. We are all unique and face different challenges and lose weight or build muscle at different rates. You might not win the prize for being the quickest or biggest loser, but you'll win something better. You are learning what works for you. You are feeling the victory when you see small changes. You are feeling more energetic when you have days that you get it right. As long as you continue to renew your purpose when you wake up, and recommit to your goals, you are headed for the winners circle.

Good habits take practice. If you give up when you are on the brink of success you will never achieve your dreams. Hang in there. Failure is only temporary. If you are speaking victory over your past addictions, you are on your way to the winners circle. You have in front of you a life time of health and fitness.

DAY 42

Good morning.

Have you noticed that how much you eat often goes up in direct proportion to how much stress you have? Funny thing about stress...it's often all about 'US'. In ten years, whatever we are stressing about today will most likely be forgotten, but today we are feeling upset so we reach for something...and something...and something.

One of the easiest ways to make the choice to move out of stress is to quit thinking of your self and how bad you feel, and see something positive in someone else. Those noisy children...give them a hug and tell them how proud you are of them. Those irritating spouses...praise them for something they've done right and quit dwelling on what they've done wrong. That pushy in-law? Find a reason to be thankful that they are in your life, and share that with them. When you practice uplifting others, you bring out the best in them. And when they are moving toward their best, your own environment becomes more serene. How nice is that.

And above all, remember that relationships are irreplaceable. Your house will be clean some day when the kids grow up. But right now is the time to enjoy them. Your honey-do list is not more important than taking a moment to reconnect and remember what you saw in each other. Finding the right dress for the occasion is less important than enjoying the occasion with the person you love. It's not about things...it's about enjoying the journey.

When you find positive in what is around you and quit dwelling on perceived wrongs happening to you, your emotional stress will lift allowing you to make good choices for your health.

DAY 43

Good morning.
 When you are struggling to transform yourself, it can
seem overwhelming to set up new habits. "Think about
your goals, pack your meals, and lay out a time to
exercise..." Be patient. Good habits will become a
lifestyle and you won't have to think after a while.

Try to keep things in perspective. When you look at that
person who has made fitness a regular part of their
lives, they don't have to struggle with it. They lay out
their gym things the night before and set the alarm for
an hour early without giving it a second thought. It is a
way of life. They throw their chicken on the George
Forman while they are eating their breakfast and pack
their lunch before they leave the house. It's no longer
something they think about...it's something they do.

When you were unhealthy your habits were not
something you thought about. You wandered into the
kitchen as soon as you got home, grabbed a bag of chips
and plopped on the couch. You mindlessly popped
Hershey kisses in your mouth as you drove to work. So,
of course, you have to think about what you are doing
now.

But every day you set a stone on the path of your
transformation. Little by little, when you build new
habits, it will become easier. Eventually you will look
back at that path of months and years and realize, it's
no big deal. It's what you do to stay fit and feel good.
And you'll be glad you started that journey.

Stick with what you are trying to accomplish. We all know there are days when we feel like our path is full of rocks. But practice will make you better. Fairly soon, the good days will outnumber the bad days. You can do this. Keep looking ahead. Keep smiling. Keep remembering that you were created to excel and you have been designed with the tools to overcome.

DAY 44

Good morning.
Those who are readers will appreciate what if feels like to find a really good book that absorbs them. Welcome to your life.

The beginning of your book may have been good or bad. You are living the adventures of those middle pages and you are the hero. It is up to you to decide how your book is going to end. Will you wither away in moaning and excuses until no one will want to read what is between the pages? Or will you, the hero, spring forward with unlimited potential, transforming yourself, impacting the lives of others around you, and living your greatest adventures?

So much about weight loss and fitness is about mindset. We live in a day when, even the poor, can get assistance to receive food. Anyone who can walk can start on a program. And at our gym we have a gentleman in a wheelchair that does killer workouts which put most people to shame. We have a lady with MS whose regular commitment to exercise inspires others around her to stay on task.

It's not about what your physical condition is. It's about making a decision to take your self to the next level, one step at a time, no matter how long it takes and no matter how many times you fall. You decide your destiny and write the ending to your story. It is your choice to be happy and thankful for your blessings. And that is not dependent on what anyone else says or does.

It is your book. You are created with awesome and unique talents that are unlike anyone else. You may be caring, you may be a great organizer, you might interact well with the elderly, and you might have a passion for music or animals. Tap into your inner talents and become the hero you were meant to be.

DAY 45

Good morning.
Every few years there is a new run of diets. For years
people avoided sugar. That nasty/wonderful stuff was
what ruined our figures. Next people avoided fat. We all
became obsessed with fat makes you fat. Then people
began reaching for gluten free. But have you noticed
that there are more fat people than ever before?

Each time a new trend comes along, the food
manufacturers rush out and create a whole new crop of
delicious processed food that our bodies do not have to
work hard to absorb and meets the criteria for our new
obsession. And yet we are fat.

When we get rid of something and process it in bulk, we
get a whole new set of chemicals to addict our bodies
too. Diet sugars, fake flavors, pretty dyes. Small wonder
our children are hyperactive and we can't concentrate,
not to mention rampant amounts of cancer and other
degenerative diseases.

Your body is a miracle of action. Cells renew, digestion
takes nutrients to all parts of your body, healing and
regeneration are a constant process. Think about how
much chance your body has to heal when you hand it
processed junk and chemicals. There was only one
person, reported, who could turn water into wine. And
that's not us. Our bodies are miraculous for what they
can do, but they cannot turn chemicals and processed
food into the vitamins, minerals, and proteins they need
to do their job.

It doesn't matter what diet you choose. Weight loss is always about calories in/calories out. However, whether your body is disease free, full of energy, and functioning at peak level can be affected greatly by whether you choose to cook your own healthy version of lasagna or buy the processed one full of sodium and over processed products. Whether you make a sandwich of whole grain, lean unprocessed meat and fresh vegetables, or whether you grab white bread and processed meat and cheese.

So here's the deal. Sugar is not bad in its natural form. An apple is full of vitamins and fiber, has a nice glycemic index (doesn't rush into your blood stream like processed sugar, and takes a while to digest), and acts like gas in your tank to give you energy.

Fat is not bad in its natural form. Nuts and avocados are good for your body. Just keep the calorie intake within your limits just like you try to do with your processed food.

So while you choose your diet to fit your lifestyle, you need to choose the foods authorized in that diet to be as unprocessed and natural as possible. That way our body has the tools to nurture and take care of us to a ripe old age.

DAY 46

Good morning.
Our body is incredible at adapting. When you have been working out for a month or more, doing the same exercises, you may find you are reaching a plateau. It's time to change what you are doing.

When you first started your cardio, you may have found it difficult to do a half hour. Now you find yourself humming along for a longer amount of time. At this point you need to kick it up. If you've been using the treadmill, try using a bike or elliptical. They all use leg muscles, but at slightly different angles. This challenges your body.

It is also time to add intensity, in bursts, to raise your metabolism and strengthen your heart, which is also a muscle. You do this by kicking up the intensity for 15-60 seconds so that you are breathing hard and the intensity is something you can do for 30 seconds that you can't do for 30 minutes (never faint or in pain). Immediately bring down the pace until your breathing evens out and you feel under control again. (This can be a short time or several minutes). When your breathing slows, kick up the intensity or pace again for 15-60 seconds and repeat the cycle. When doing intervals like this, you can work out for less time, because you are working harder. A half hour workout can now be over in 20 minutes. And because you are getting your heart pumping and blood moving to all parts of your body, you will raise your metabolism for the next 24 hours and send healing nutrients to your muscles.

Likewise you need to change up your weight lifting. If you are using machines, try cables or free weights that use muscles from a different angle or involve using your stabilizing helper muscles. If you are pyramiding up or down in weight, try volume or power moves. Try to plan workouts that use a combination of muscles, or those side muscles that you never seem to exercise. (Most exercises are done in forward motion...biking, hiking, lifting weights...Your body is three dimensional and needs muscles worked from the side and three-quarter angles also.) Remember that when you are pushing a set of muscles to exhaustion by adding weight, you are creating tiny muscle tears. Let these muscles rest for 3-5 days while you work out a different set of muscles.

And finally... make sure your nutrition adapts to meet your changing lifestyle. Weight loss is about calories in/calories out, but when you cut your calories too low, your body will try to adapt by conserving its resources. You will have less energy to do good workouts and drag through your day. This is your body lowering your metabolism to conserve energy in what it thinks is a time of starvation. You can tweak your diet by using slightly less calories for a couple of days and then a higher calorie day to fool your body into thinking there is no deprivation intended.

Or you may actually need a few more high nutrition calories to keep your body functioning at the high level it needs for intense workouts which will build muscle and burn fat. This is where you have to think about how you feel and what is healthy to meet your goals.

DAY 47

Good morning.
Ever have a moment when you just want to cry? When you wonder, "What is wrong with me? Why can't I get this right? What happened to me today or this weekend?" Take a deep breath. Have patience.

Every great artist or professional has moments of discouragement. That's part of the learning process. Ever heard someone learning to play an instrument? I'm sure every mom out there who had a kid practicing their notes, will remember the wincing and trauma to their ears as they watched the painful process of learning to read music. It takes practice and practice and practice and anyone will tell you a LOT of wrong notes before the player can HEAR and discern the path their fingers need to take, to get it right. Then as each day compounds on the next, there comes a day when that same mom is sitting in the audience with tears of pride streaming down her face as her child plays beautiful music.

Your body is your instrument. You may have days when you play a lot of wrong notes trying to figure out what works best to play beautiful music. It takes determination and grit to keep going through all the wincing and bad times to teach the body to consistently reach for the good notes that makes it hum along in tune. You may be grinding along at 'Twinkle Twinkle Little Star' right now, but eventually you'll be sailing through Mozart. The exercise program will be habit. Reaching for healthy alternatives and making your own meals will become the norm. You will be an athlete.

Being an athlete happens in the mind. When you have done so many workouts that you would feel bad if you skipped your workout, when you are so used to cooking your giant pan of meatloaf for the week and prepping your veggies that you would wonder what you'd eat if you didn't get it done, then you have become an athlete. Your body may not have lost all the weight it needs to or built all the muscle you desire, but once your mind has made the switch, your body has no other choice than to follow.

In the meantime, every workout you put in takes you closer to that change over. Every time you prep a meal, it makes those bad days take a step lower on the ladder rung of your life. There will come a day when you will be emotional and go for a run instead of a donut. There will be a time when you forget your lunch and stop at the store for an apple and a slice of baked chicken instead of going through the drive through. You got this! Believe!

DAY 48

Good morning.
What do you think is a dieter's biggest downfall? Is it
the bacon double cheeseburger with fries? Actually,
soda ranks highest in the average diet. Loaded with
sugar and caffeine it goes through your body quickly
and leaves you wanting more.

And for those who are fighting weight... that yummy,
cool, refreshing diet coke, that you feel is saving you
calories, may not be your best friend after all. Diet
sweeteners have the potential to cause kidney problems.
They can disrupt your body's ability to regulate calorie
intake because the body reads the product as being
sweet, but gets no food value from the source of
sweetness.

Dieters who consume just one or two diet soda's each
day have up to a 500% larger waistline, and often have
cravings and overeating problems beyond what the non-
diet soda drinkers have. Diet sodas usually contain
types of preservatives that regular soda's do not. These
preservatives inhibit mold and cause severe cell damage
to the DNA in the mitochondria. Soft drink cans are
coated with a substance (BPA) that has been linked to
everything from heart disease, to reproductive problems,
to obesity. The PH level of diet coke leads to a much
higher incidence of tooth decay. Overall, the negative
consequences of drinking diet coke far outweigh the
temporary satisfaction of a cold, non-calorie drink.

Energy drinks do not rate much better. Sugar and caffeine are often the primary delivery system of energy. Many times the additional herbs are not high enough to do much more than add to the label. And because the sources of those herbs are not regulated in energy drinks, they can come from sources that irradiate, use contaminated water, or use toxic pesticides. This can lead to harmful toxins in our bodies. Energy drinks can raise blood pressure, be addictive (caffeine), disrupt sleep patterns, and aggravate psychiatric conditions. Too much caffeine can lead to vomiting, a fast heart rate, seizure, and even death.

Realistically a person should examine why they are reaching for these drinks. Are you sleep deprived? Are you getting enough exercise and good nutrition to have the energy you need? Are you drinking enough water to avoid being dehydrated? Is it just a habit to reach for something that has flavor to it? It may be time to re-evaluate your priorities in your life, add a regular source of good old fashioned water, and rearrange your schedule to get the workouts and sleep your body needs.

DAY 49

Good morning.
I had a wonderful friend, who is very heavy, approach
me about going to the gym. She was worried about
feeling awkward and embarrassed to work out in front
of others. She was afraid people would stare or talk
about her. This woman works at a fast food restaurant.
Does she not think people notice when a woman who is
80 pounds overweight hands them their fries?

Here's the thing. Everybody becomes comfortable in the
environment they are used to. You may not like how you
look at work, going to the grocery store, and doing
errands. You do them anyway, regardless of what people
think, because it's necessary.

If you are exhausted walking to the end of the block,
that gym is necessary. It's where you can build some
muscle to reshape your body and burn up that fat. It's a
safe environment where you can start a cardio program
and work at your pace until you are stronger. Get over
the idea that people are watching you. They are doing
their own workouts and all of them started from
somewhere that involved the gym to meet a need in their
life.

Some of those people in the gym have lost massive
amounts of weight. They are not there to mock you.
They may be your best support system and source of
ideas to help you reach your goal. The gym is not full of
skinny babes and muscle heads. That was the days of
the steroids.

Gyms are full of normal people of all ages who want the energy and strength to make it through their work day and need stamina to raise their kids in the midst of a life that bombards them with fast food and sugar. They go to a gym to tone and lose weight. They go to the gym to be healthy. They go to release tension and have time away from the stress of their lives. They are people of all shapes and sizes who are making a difference in their lives one day at a time.

Realistically, you may be awkward when you walk into a gym because it is a new environment to you. Within a few days you will feel at home and relaxed in your new routine.

You will get much more positive attention being a heavy person who is in a gym doing something about it, then being a heavy person handing someone a bag of fries or walking through the grocery store with a cart full of cookies. Think about what is really important to you; A few uncomfortable moments of newness, or a lifetime of regret and tears. Soon, you could be the one at work who is full of energy and showing an example to all the other workers who are waddling through life too embarrassed to join a gym.

DAY 50

Good morning.
Many people equate detoxifying the body with fasting.
This doesn't have to be the case. Our bodies are
designed to heal and work efficiently. When we spend
years weighing ourselves down with toxins in our
environment, our bodies can become sluggish and tired
(not to mention retaining weight).

Part of eating clean is allowing our liver and organs to
effectively get rid of the bad bacteria and toxins in our
bodies and build the good bacteria, that keeps us
healthy. A detox diet will create conditions that will help
the body get rid of excess fat, heal better, and have more
energy.

Here are some of the key detox foods to keep your body
humming along:
>   Green leafy vegetables (fiber and feeds the good
>   bacteria)
>   Cold water fish (Has less toxins, has good fats and
>   proteins)
>   Free range chickens (No hormones)
>   Berries (Kills cravings and has fiber)
>   Apple Cider Vinegar (promotes hydrocloric acid
>   and helps digestion)
>   Lemon Water
>   Plant based protein powder (For people who eat
>   little or no meat).
>   Herbal teas (boost energy)
>   Unsweetened coconut milk and/or coconut oil
>   (good oil, smaller/shorter fats)
>   Lots and lots of water

You can create shakes, casseroles, and other dishes
from combinations of these foods.

Foods to eliminate from our diets while detoxing:
>   Soy
>   Processed sugar

Alcohol/coffee/soda
Beef/pork
Creamed veggies
Dairy/Eggs
Peanuts (Can have fungi on them)
Gluten

When you are first eliminating foods from your diet, you may experience some headaches and side effects.

After you have done a period of time on the detox diet, you can add foods that have good nutritional value back to your diet. The foods listed to add or avoid are about helping the liver get back into optimum condition to keep your body healthy.

When losing weight, it is always about creating a program that you can live with long term to stay lean and healthy. Sometimes taking a week or two to detox your body and then moving back into your own healthy eating program using foods you prefer, will help your body with it's ability to do the work it was created to do.

DAY 51

Good morning.
We've all had friends who seem to continually struggle.
Things always seem to be going wrong for them. Have
you ever listened to the words that come out of their
mouths? "I'm tired today. Today is going to be a long,
hard day. I'm so depressed. My kids exhaust me. I hate
my job. I can't find a job. I can't lose any weight. I can't
seem to stay on an exercise program..." Those people are
creating their future. They are setting themselves up for
failure, in that area of their life, by the words from their
mouth.

When we say something out loud, our own ears hear
our message and our bodies react to them. Want to be
fat and miserable the rest of your life? Just keep saying,
"I hate myself. I'm so fat! I can't stay on a diet." You are
guaranteeing yourself a life of what you believe.

It's important to talk blessings into your future whether
your body and life is at that point or not. A person who
is sick will heal slower and stay sick longer when they
talk about feeling ill and unwell. The person who says
they never getting sick, and that they never stay down
long, is staying healthy and healed through mental
direction. Their body is following the message that their
mind is sending.

When a person is moaning about not being able to get a
job, their heads are down like an ostrich in the sand.
They can't see a door that might be open, they don't give
positive interviews, and they stop searching effectively.
The result is that they sabotage their own success with
their constant talk of not being able to find a job. It is
important to speak positive about that better job coming
to them, to eagerly seek out interviews and be open to
that job that didn't seem to be much, opening into a
much better opportunity.

When you are heavy and out of shape, it is important for you to speak blessings into your life. "I am getting fitter every day. I look for opportunities to work out. I enjoy foods that make my body feel well and build health and energy. I am free of addictions and becoming healthier every day. I am strong enough to stick to a workout program. I am motivated to exercise and eat right each day."

We are blessed with the ability to have choices. You have the strength, intelligence, and ability to create a life of abundance and happiness beyond anything you've seen. You have not lived your best day yet. You have not reached your highest potential yet. Your future is as easy as making the choice to speak negative or positive words into your life.

DAY 52

Good morning.
Most people know how important it is to exercise and eat right. What is often overlooked, in a fitness program, is the importance of stretching. Most people tend to skimp or skip this step, preferring to jump right in to the meaty part of our work outs, with the feeling that they don't have time to stretch or it bores them. Stretching can be as important as any other component of your program.

It is now recognized that, if you are going to be doing an extremely heavy or taxing workout, stretching right before your work out can reduce the amount of load you can push your muscles through. This doesn't mean you can't stretch. Active stretching involves doing actions that are going to mimic your activity, before you begin the activity, to warm the muscle. For instance...you can do lunges before running or throw a ball against the wall from chest level prior to doing chest presses.

And because you are planning a heavy workout later in the day, doesn't mean you can't do static stretching (holding a stretch for 30 seconds) before your workout. It just means you need to do your pre-stretching at least an hour prior to your work-out. Most people in our society clearly need an ongoing stretching program that is done daily, regardless of whether you exercise that day or not. This is to counteract the muscle imbalances you create with your lifestyle.

For example...If your feet turn outward, the muscles on that side of your leg are stronger than the muscles on the inside of your leg. Over time, because the foot is turned out, the muscles on that side of the leg become shorter because there is less distance to pull with the foot turned out. The muscles on the inside of the leg are stretched further because they are weaker and can't hold the foot in a straight forward position.

It is necessary to do a continual stretching program to allow those outside muscles to lengthen so that your foot can walk straight. Now you can do resistance exercise in the gym for the inside of your leg to make it as strong as the outside, enabling you to walk with your feet straight. A day or two of stretching for a few moments, once or twice a week, will not eliminate the imbalanced muscles in your leg that you have built through constantly walking around with your feet turned out. You need to be on a consistent routine of stretching.

These muscle imbalances can be tracked to your lifestyle. If you sit in a chair or on a couch for long periods of time, there is a good chance that the muscles on the front side of your body are becoming shorter and tighter than the muscles along your back. Stretching that involves standing up and leaning backward will help counterbalance the constant leaning forward position.

It is fairly easy to get into a habit of stretching each time you get up and move around. Stretches to counterbalance muscle imbalances need to be held for approximately 30 seconds to feel a stretching sensation, but never pain. After 20-30 seconds your body will soften a little and you will be able to take the stretch slightly deeper, again without pain. Then release.

Look at your body in the mirror. If your shoulders round forward, then the front of you (chest, front of shoulders) needs to stretch backward daily. Then exercises that strengthen your upper back and the back of your shoulders need to be added to your routine to make those muscles strong enough to hold your posture straight.

For most of us, it's as simple as pin pointing what is tight and stretching it out, then strengthening the opposite side. If you continue through life with muscle imbalances, the pressure of using your body without being in alignment can eventually cause injuries and further imbalances.

After your workout, it is equally important to stretch those muscles that you used. These muscles are warm and respond to static stretching. By doing the same 30 second hold in a stretching position, that doesn't involve pain, you can increase your flexibility and lengthen your muscles.

Done daily, your range of motion will increase and muscles will stay balanced and ready for the next hard workout. Muscles that stay long and flexible will have less chance of you over reaching your range of motion and tearing something.

Overall, it is important to recognize the benefits of stretching and add a daily dose to your lifestyle. Whether you do your stretches when you first roll out of bed or at the gym... your body will thank you with years of better posture and less chance of injury.

DAY 53

Good morning.

If you were facing a catastrophic disaster... your home was sweeping away, a fire was engulfing your area, a tornado was tearing every obstacle out of its path...what would you reach for first? Would you try to save your favorite quilt? Would you grab your favorite pictures? Or would you reach for the living objects around you...people and animals. It has been seen over and over again the heroism of people reaching out to save someone in extreme danger in spite of the potential danger to themselves.

Now let's narrow that down a bit. If your boat capsized and your child and your neighbors child were drowning... which child would you reach for first? It is very humbling to many of us who claim to love everyone equally to realized that in that moment when the brain can't over think, make excuses, and analyze things to death, that your immediate reaction would be to save your own child. Let's face it...most parents would give their own life to save the life of their child. We spend years feeding our children, making sure they are warm, getting them to the doctor, off to school, and trying to help them mature.

So why do we feed them sugar? We don't feed them cocaine. Why do we teach them to read, but we don't take the time to teach them to exercise and take care of their bodies? We are examples to those around us. Our children, our friends, and our families need good examples to know how to be healthy themselves.

I realize that each one of us need to make a choice to be healthy ourselves. It is our journey. But if you take the time to look at those you love most, can't you use the pain of what you are doing to them to motivate you to keep going? They can be your biggest reason to not give up. To keep trying until you succeed.

It doesn't matter how many times you've fallen. The example is that we keep getting back on the path and moving forward. We don't give up. We practice a lifestyle that will take us into a happy and healthy old age.

There is not one of us who want to live longer than our children. So we certainly do not want to build obesity and degenerative disease into our children through bad nutrition and unhealthy lifestyle. Our children need to see us being positive, even when we fall, and getting back on the fitness path. How can they succeed if we do not believe success is possible?

The example, we share, is that we are each created with a different combination of abilities and talents and that our gift, from our creator, is the special, wonderful person that we are. Our gift, back to our creator, is what we do with what he has given us.

DAY 54

Good morning.
Today you will have 24 hours to work with. That is not very much when you consider what you need to get done today. But it is no more time than anyone else has.

"I don't have time to exercise", is consistently a top excuse for not working out. The reality here is that the body isn't lazy...the mind is. It's too hot. It's too cold. I'm too tired. I have too much to do. I'll start tomorrow. Sound like anyone you know?

This is where you, getting up every day and retraining your mind, comes in to play. If you have a vision board, you look at your goals and try to absorb the pleasure you will feel meeting your goals. You verbally tell yourself out loud that doors are opening, blessings are coming to you daily, and you have the ability to eat right and exercise today. Then do it. Ignore the voice in your head that says you are too tired, and get moving. Getting up an hour early to exercise wont' kill you, but being obese might.

Most of us can do something for a day that would seem overwhelming for a life time. You only have to approach your fitness one day at a time. And for that day, be the best you can be.

DAY 55

Good morning.
Many of us would love to run a successful company and
call the shots. Hello. You do. You are the president of
the company of "YOU". You are the owner, the CEO, the
high hauncho, the boss. What you say goes in the
company of YOU".

Like any great company, there needs to be a vision. A
way you want your company to look and function. And
there needs to be an operating plan to take that
business to the top. You wouldn't start a business, then
check out for several years and expect it to flourish and
grow.

When you first start growing a business, you put in a lot
of personal time. You make it your priority. You think
about strategies and deadlines. You set goals. Later on,
when the business is humming along where you want it
to be, you can take an occasional vacation and step
back in without much problem. But in the early days of
growing a business you need to be there to correct any
downfalls. You need to pay attention to anything that
isn't working and substitute another plan of attack. You
need to have a weekly staff meeting, assess what works
and what doesn't and evolve as you see the need. You
will need to decide when your company closes down and
sleeps, when it is time for meal breaks, and when it is
'working out' hours. You will own the company of "YOU"
for the rest of your life, 24 hours a day, and 7 days a
week. If you can take care of this company, you can do
anything.
 But if you check out and ignore your company. If you
take an extended vacation, allow lunch hours to run
into each other, let the work out week dwindle to
nothing...your company will eventually fail. You would
not take a business that you'd only operated about 7
weeks and say, "Golly, I should be at the top by now. I'll
just give up".

Where you put your time and energy, you will succeed. What you ignore and let slide will fail. Take a moment and look at the company of "YOU". This is your chance to take a company that is teetering and change its course. This is where you can shine. It can be your greatest achievement.

DAY 56

Good Morning.
So what exactly is a cheat meal used for? To help you be
successful at your weight loss or maintenance. No one
can stay on a diet forever. Those people who are
successful have created a fitness lifestyle that takes into
account that they may have a sweet tooth, or the
thought of never eating biscuits and gravy again sends
them into a spiral of depression. That's why diets don't
work, and lifestyles do.

On a diet, you create a mentality of despair. "I can never
have chocolate again," or, "I can only eat this disgusting
plate of broccoli when I'd rather eat macaroni and
cheese" So when you break your diet, you eat every
yummy food you can think of, knowing you will deprive
yourself tomorrow.

If you incorporate a cheat meal into your fitness plan,
you can now use this to stay successful. "I choose to eat
nutritious this week, because on Sunday I will get to
have biscuits and gravy for breakfast. And the following
week I can do the same thing or change it to something
else". You can look ahead at your week and choose the
day and meal you want to cheat on. "I can eat healthy
now, because on Thursday I'm going to a birthday party
and I want to enjoy having cake" Here's the beauty of
the cheat meal.

Most people break their diets and feel bad the whole
time. They beat themselves up and take the enjoyment
out of their treat. When you give yourself permission to
eat what you want for one meal, you can relish and
enjoy it, knowing that one bad meal in a week of good
meals is not going to send your fitness lifestyle in the
wrong direction.

If you have the chronic diet mentality of breaking your diet and spiraling into a binge, this may take some practice. You will have to reset your thought patterns to relax and enjoy the journey.

If you have a sugar addiction, you may need to forgo the cheat meal a month to allow your body to get away from the sugar and learn to enjoy wholesome food. But if you know that cheat meal is there ready to enjoy, when and where you choose to use it, you can begin to recover from your yo yo dieting, where you feel you must be on the top following your diet perfectly, or lying at the bottom eating everything in sight, with no middle ground.

The point of having a fitness lifestyle is to be able to live our life fully. We want to avoid feeling like we are missing out on everything we love in order to be healthy.

DAY 57

Good morning.

Have you heard people say that creating a habit takes 21-30 days? Yep. That's why we want to pack our lunches EVERY DAY. It's why we want to drink water when we get up, 1/2 hour before and 1/2 hour after every meal, and before bedtime EVERY DAY. It's why we want to exercise EVERY day, even if your day off, from working out, is a relaxing walk.

So here's what you might not realize...When you start doing something different, your body resists the new routine. After a month, you may have established a new habit, and your body may have quit groaning about having to do it, but you haven't convinced it that this way is better than the old way. It's still deciding. It's just as easy for your body to take the old path as it is to take the new path.

Once you get approximately two months into the new routine, your body actually begins to like and prefer the new routine over the old one. So when you are trying to transform yourself it's important to stick with a new habit until it really does stick. That's why a two month weight loss/fitness program is a good time span. It's long enough to create positive results without the boredom and feeling of being overwhelmed that a longer amount of time can create.

After that couple of months, it's time to tweak what you are doing, set some new goals, and create a few more great habits.

DAY 58

Good morning.
Are you one of those people who get disgusted with themselves, hate how they look and feel, have no energy...and start a new diet? And how do you go about doing that diet? Most of us decide, "That's it! I'm going to stop eating sugar, drink a gallon of water every day, exercise seven days a week for two hours a day, cook every meal at home, take my vitamins and supplements every day, stop smoking, and never touch carbs again. Oh, and while I'm at it, I'll cut down my calories to between 800 and 1200 calories and get that weight, that I've packed on for 15 years, off in 30 days!"

So how is that working for you? There are a few who do really well at jumping into a project and using the momentum to push them selves along. For the majority of us, our body reacts by going into survival mode: "You're killing me, man! You're killing me! I'm not used to eating this healthy crap! I'm giving you a head ache. What do you mean I can't have soda? That's what my blood is made of! No Sugar! Are you insane! I need my drug man! I need my drug man! Give me! Give me!"

For many of us, a few concrete goals are much more attainable. If you eat 3500 calories a day, it will be easier for you cut down to 2500 calories for a month and concentrate on a few healthier choices to keep your body from going into diet behavior and rebelling. Then you can cut your calories again the next month to keep moving forward toward your goal. Remember that past experience has shown that you can't live on a diet forever, and if you blow it, you will be likely to balloon up worse than before. If you decided to concentrate on drinking 10 glasses of water this month, then next month retain that shaky new habit and add 3 days of week exercising, then retain that habit and the next month cut out going to the fast food place 6 of the 7 days in a week, you will begin to see lasting changes that become a lifestyle of fitness.

What you've done to your body didn't happen over night. If you haven't been successful trying to cram your weight loss efforts into a month time frame, back off a bit, set a more realistic time schedule, and move at a pace your body can handle. With patience and a positive attitude you can create the lifestyle you dream of.

DAY 59

Good morning.
One part of fitness is your physical exercise. That gives
you that great boost of energy, self-esteem, and ability
to take care of your body. The other part of fitness is
your mind. If you have no way to de-stress, unwind,
or renew your spirit, it can spill over into emotional
eating and despair.

Think about what gives you that 'ah' moment that
makes your world feel right. This can be painting,
writing in a journal, biking, training your dog, taking a
bath, walking, meditating, yoga, listening to music,
reading a good book, etc... This is where you want to
start your day. If you need to set your alarm and paint
for a 1/2 hour to start your day feeling renewed, or sit
outside and watch the sunrise, then make it part of
your lifestyle. If your hobby or feel good action, is not
exercise, you can now follow your plan to get in a good
exercise session for the day, pack your meals, etc. and
move into your day on a positive note.

If we don't build a few moments of 'me' time into your
lifestyle, you risk drowning in everyday pressure.
Sometimes the best medicine, that can be prescribed, is
letting everyone else take care of themselves for a few
minutes, so you can take care of yourself. This isn't
selfish. It's survival. It makes you a more balanced
person, it makes you calmer and happier, it allows you
to re-strengthen your inner stamina to be a better mom,
dad, spouse, parent, etc. It rebuilds your endurance to
reach out and live your life with passion and follow your
dreams.

Like taking care of a car, we all know that making sure
you have a fully charged battery will take you much
further on your journey, than a battery that is nearly
depleated.

DAY 60

Good morning,
When you can see the end in sight, it is time to be thinking where you are going next. One of the great tragedies that can happen is that when we finish our self-made goal, we no longer have the drive to push forward. It is easy at that point to fall into old habits and gain our weight back.

Whether you have been strong the entire challenge or whether you have had some rough patches, it is important to continue pressing toward the end goal. Big or little changes, your self-worth needs to keep doing your best so that you finish the time frame you set for yourself and don't feel like you gave up...again. Commit to finishing strong and start thinking about what you will be doing next.

Fitness is a lifestyle, not a short term solution. If you've lost the weight you set out to lose, you may want to think about starting a jogging program after you finish your challenge, with a 5k in mind. You might want to revamp your weight training and tightening program with a vacation as your next goal. You might want to set a new goal to start a biking program and take a tour somewhere. You might want to get some certification and become a trainer in some type of class. Or you might want to rest and hold the weight you are at for a week or so (without gaining anything back), then start a new weight loss challenge to bring yourself closer to your goal.

Whatever you do, you do not want to slide into old habits and those familiar feelings of self-disgust. You have the rest of your life in front of you. How exciting is that! Don't waste one moment of it bogged down in junk food and lack of energy. Go out and LIVE.

LET'S EVALUATE YOUR PROGRESS. Don't shy away from taking an honest look at yourself now. Remember that your body is in a constant state of change and renewal. If you are not heavier, you are successful. If you lost even a few pounds of fat, you are successful. If you are drinking more water, you are successful. If you are eating home cooked food and packing your own meals, you are more successful. If you are more careful to take your supplements, you are successful. If you have a more positive mindset, if you get back in the game when you fall short, if you are reaching out to others, if you are exercising more, if you are setting goals.....any and all are signs of success.

If you have done nothing more than get determined to not give up, then you have figured out the real secret to success. There is nothing more important than 'not quitting'. That is the strength of the human race. We are all fearfully and wonderfully created. We will all reach our goals in our own timeline that is different from everyone else.

So no matter how you think you've done, reweigh and measure yourself. This is your guideline for the next month. This is the starting point for a whole new set of goals to keep moving forward.

If you had trouble in any area, figure out what tripped you up and set out a whole new plan of action. Make yourself a vision board. Download yourself some motivational music. Find a motivational picture. Plan your meals. Plan your exercise. When you are 90 years of age, you want to say, "I don't have a bucket list and I don't have any regrets. I've lived my life with passion!"

If you need to keep going with your fitness journey, start back at the beginning of the book and begin again. Staying motivated is about continually putting in positive and changing out the negative.

www.ingramcontent.com/pod-product-compliance
Lightning Source LLC
Chambersburg PA
CBHW072248310526
45795CB00011B/473